Handbook of
REHABILITATION MEDICINE

Handbook of
REHABILITATION MEDICINE

Editor

KONG Keng He

Department of Rehabilitation Medicine
Tan Tock Seng Hospital, Singapore

Co-editors

YAP Giok Mei Samantha
LOH Yong Joo

Department of Rehabilitation Medicine
Tan Tock Seng Hospital, Singapore

Tan Tock Seng
HOSPITAL

World Scientific

Published by

World Scientific Publishing Co. Pte. Ltd.

5 Toh Tuck Link, Singapore 596224

USA office: 27 Warren Street, Suite 401-402, Hackensack, NJ 07601

UK office: 57 Shelton Street, Covent Garden, London WC2H 9HE

Library of Congress Cataloging-in-Publication Data
Names: Kong, Keng He, editor. | Yap, Samantha Giok Mei, editor. | Loh, Yong Joo, editor.
Title: Handbook of rehabilitation medicine / Keng He Kong, Samantha Giok Mei Yap,
    Yong Joo Loh.
Description: New Jersey : World Scientific, 2016. |
    Includes bibliographical references and index.
Identifiers: LCCN 2016032950| ISBN 9789813148703 (hardcover : alk. paper) |
    ISBN 9789813148710 (pbk. : alk. paper)
Subjects: | MESH: Rehabilitation | Handbooks
Classification: LCC RD795 | NLM WB 39 | DDC 617/.03--dc23
LC record available at https://lccn.loc.gov/2016032950

British Library Cataloguing-in-Publication Data
A catalogue record for this book is available from the British Library.

Artist: Lionel Seow

Preface

Rehabilitation Medicine is the field of medicine that seeks to restore function in individuals with disabilities. It enables the disabled and is unique as it transcends specificity of age and disease. Good functional outcomes are best achieved through interdisciplinary teamwork which addresses the multifaceted needs of the individual. This handbook is the culmination of effort from my colleagues at the Department of Rehabilitation Medicine, Tan Tock Seng Hospital. The Department of Rehabilitation Medicine is the first Rehabilitation Medicine department in Singapore and for many years, has been instrumental in the training of rehabilitation physicians (and other rehabilitation professionals) and shaping of practice of rehabilitation.

It is not the intention of this handbook to be comprehensive or exhaustive. Rather, it seeks to address common rehabilitation conditions in a practical, problem-based manner. Thus, included are chapters on rehabilitation of stroke, spinal cord injury, traumatic brain injury and lower limb amputation. Also included are Rehabilitation in the Intensive Care Unit and Rehabilitation Technology, two areas which the department is actively growing and developing.

I would like to take this opportunity to express my gratitude to two persons. The first is the late Dr Tan Eng Seng, former head of Department of Rehabilitation Medicine, Tan Tock Seng Hospital. An amiable and optimistic person, he convinced me of the future of Rehabilitation Medicine as a specialty when I first joined the department in 1991, and he was right. The second person is my good friend and colleague, Dr Chan Kay Fei, with whom I have journeyed, through thick and thin, in this field for the last 25 years.

And finally, to all my patients, past and present, a big thank you. You have been my best teachers, in the field of Rehabilitation Medicine and in the lessons of life.

KONG Keng He
Adjunct Associate Professor
National University of Singapore
Yong Loo Lin School of Medicine

Senior Consultant
Department of Rehabilitation Medicine
Tan Tock Seng Hospital, Singapore

List of Contributors

CHAN Kay Fei, MBBS, MRCP
Senior Consultant, Rehabilitation Medicine

CHAN Wai Lim William, MBBS, FAFRM (RACP)
Senior Consultant, Rehabilitation Medicine

CHUA Sui Geok Karen, MBBS, FRCP
Senior Consultant, Rehabilitation Medicine

KIM Jongmoon, MD
Consultant, Rehabilitation Medicine

KONG Keng He, MBBS, MRCP
Senior Consultant, Rehabilitation Medicine

LIM Pang Hung, MSc (Physiotherapy)
Principal Physiotherapist, Rehabilitation Medicine

LOH Yong Joo, MBBS, MRCP
Consultant, Rehabilitation Medicine

LUI Wen Li, MBBS, MRCP
Senior Resident, Rehabilitation Medicine

NEO Jong Jong, MBBS, FAFRM (RACP)
Consultant, Rehabilitation Medicine

PALANIAPPAN K, MBBS, MRCP
Consultant, Rehabilitation Medicine

RAJESWARAN Deshan Kumar, MBBS, MRCP
Consultant, Rehabilitation Medicine

RATHA KRISHNAN Rathi, MBBS, MPH
Senior Resident Physician, Rehabilitation Medicine

SETIOTA Nuez Odessa, MD
Senior Resident Physician, Rehabilitation Medicine

List of Contributors

TAN En-Xian Emily, MBBS, MRCP
Senior Resident, Rehabilitation Medicine

TAN Ping Ping, MBBS, MRCP
Consultant, Rehabilitation Medicine

TJAN Soon Yin, MBBS, MRCP
Head & Senior Consultant, Rehabilitation Medicine

TOH Ee Mui Shirlene, Diploma Health Science
(Occupational Therapy), Master of Health Science
Principal Occupational Therapist, Rehabilitation Medicine

TOW Peh Er Adela, MBBS, MRCP
Senior Consultant, Rehabilitation Medicine

VADASSERY Shaji Jose, MBBS, MRCP
Consultant, General Medicine

VICTOR Somu, MBBS
Senior Resident Physician, Rehabilitation Medicine

WONG Chin Jung, MBBS, MRCP
Associate Consultant, Rehabilitation Medicine

YAP Eng Ching, MBBS, MRCP
Senior Consultant, Rehabilitation Medicine

YAP Giok Mei Samantha, MBBS, MRCP
Senior Consultant, Rehabilitation Medicine

YEN Hwee Ling, MBBS, FRCP
Consultant, Rehabilitation Medicine

ZENG Shanyong, MBBS
Senior Resident, Rehabilitation Medicine

*All contributors are from Tan Tock Seng Hospital, Singapore

Contents

Preface v

List of Contributors vii

1 Functional Assessment in
Rehabilitation Medicine...........................1

2 Deconditioning and Immobility
in Hospitalised Patients...........................9

3 Stroke Rehabilitation.............................15

4 Spinal Cord Injury Rehabilitation 31

5 Traumatic Brain Injury
Rehabilitation..49

6 Geriatric Rehabilitation...........................61

7 Lower Limb Amputee Rehabilitation:
Basic Grounding 75

8 Cardiopulmonary
Rehabilitation..85

9 Rehabilitation of Low Back Pain.............93

10 Rehabilitation Approach to Common
Cancer-related Problems 101

Contents

11 Adult Joint Reconstruction
Rehabilitation.......................................111

12 Rehabilitation in the Intensive
Care Unit 133

13 Pain issues in the
Rehabilitation Patient Population—
a Systems Approach 141

14 Practical Approach
to Spasticity...147

15 Medical Emergencies and
Complications in Rehabilitation 159

16 Walking Aids and Lower
Limb Orthotics 177

17 Upper Limb Assistive Devices and
Wheelchair Prescription 187

18 Rehabilitation Technology 193

19 Acupuncture in Rehabilitation 205

1

Functional Assessment in Rehabilitation Medicine

CHAN Wai Lim William

Introduction

Rehabilitation medicine is the specialty focusing on the optimisation of functions lost in diseases and injuries.

Functional assessment is an extension of the conventional medical history taking and physical examination. It goes beyond the identification of the foci and the extent of the disease, disorder or injury of the patient, and includes all levels of disability specific to the patient.

The term "disability" as defined by the World Health Organisation (WHO) encompasses all levels of functional losses, which are systematically catalogued in the International Classification of Functioning, Disability and Health (ICF). ICF offers an international, scientific tool shifting from a purely medical model to a bio-psycho-social model of human functioning and disability. The three domains of functioning are defined as:

1. **Impairments:** any loss or abnormality of body structure or of physiological or psychological function

2. **Activity Limitations:** the nature and extent of functioning at the level of the person

3. **Participation Restrictions:** the nature and extent of a person's involvement in life situations in relationship to impairments, activities, health conditions, and contextual factors

Source: ICF Website: http://www.who.int/classifications/icf/en/

Health Condition

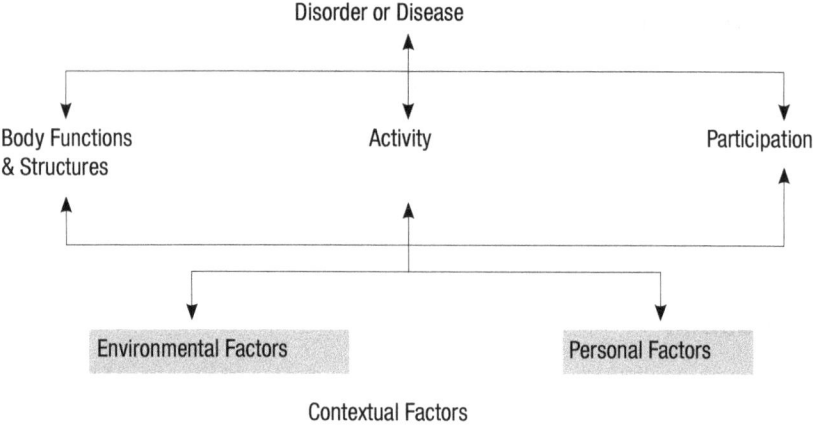

Disorder or Disease

Body Functions
& Structures

Activity

Participation

Environmental Factors

Personal Factors

Contextual Factors

Fig. 1. The ICF Model of Disability.

Rehabilitation medicine functional assessment

Apart from the assessment of the primary impairments caused by the disease or injury, the functional assessment must explore potential secondary impairments in other systems.

For example, for a patient with a pure motor stroke, apart from thorough assessment of the motor impairments, symptoms and signs of common secondary impairments such as shoulder pain and subluxation, venous thrombo-embolism and spasticity must be explored and documented. Furthermore, symptoms and signs of activity limitations and participation restrictions such as ability to perform self-care activities and use of public transport must also be evaluated.

Table 1. The essential elements of the Rehabilitation Medical Functional Assessment.

Component	Examples
History taking	
History of present illness	Location, onset, quality, severity, duration, modifying factors, context, associated symptoms, course of all symptoms, and medical management to date.

	For disabilities as a result of accident or injury—details of circumstances surrounding the incident.
Functional history	• Basic Activities of Daily Living (BADL):
	▪ Self-care: bathing, personal hygiene, grooming, toileting, dressing, eating
	▪ Mobility: bed mobility, transfers, ambulation, stair climbing, wheelchair mobility, assistive device usage
	• Instrumental ADL: meal preparation, laundry, use of communication devices, home maintenance, personal health management, financial management, driving, shopping, care of others, including pets, etc.
	• Cognition
	• Communication
Past medical history	• Specific conditions such as cardiovascular, musculoskeletal, rheumatological, pulmonary and neurological conditions which may lead to pre-morbid disabilities
	• Medications
Social history	Home environment, living circumstances, family and friends support system, domestic helper, usual modes of transport, vocational history, recreational activities and hobbies, spirituality, litigation, insurance and compensation issues.
Family history	As related to the presenting illness.
Review of systems	In particular, enquire on symptoms associated with secondary impairments as a result of immobilisation, de-conditioning, weakness, sensory loss, autonomic dysfunction and pain.

Physical examination

General	• Cardiac
	• Pulmonary
	• Abdominal
	• Others
Neurological	• General
	■ Level of consciousness
	■ Attention
	■ Orientation
	■ Memory
	■ General knowledge
	■ Abstract thinking
	■ Insight and judgement
	■ Mood and affect
	• Communication
	• Cranial nerve examination
	• Sensation
	• Motor control
	■ Involuntary movements
	■ Tone
	■ Strength
	■ Coordination
	■ Praxis
	• Reflexes
	■ Superficial
	■ Deep
	■ Primitive

Musculoskeletal	<ul><li>Inspection<ul><li>Behaviour</li><li>Physical symmetry</li><li>Joint deformity etc.</li></ul></li><li>Palpation<ul><li>Joint stability</li><li>Range of motion (active, passive)</li><li>Painful joints and muscles</li><li>Strength testing (Manual Muscle Testing)</li></ul></li><li>Joint-specific provocative manoeuvres</li></ul>

Assessment of activity limitations and participation restrictions

General	Based on information gathered above, summarise the impact of all the impairments in the person's activities and participations.

Functional measurements

"If you cannot measure it, you cannot improve it."

**Lord Kelvin
(Sir William Thomson)**

Many functional assessment measurement tools have been developed to quantify the extent of impairments, activity limitations and participation restrictions.

These tools can also serve to monitor progress and track improvements in function.

The choice of scales used in various rehabilitation setting depends on the patient profile of the rehabilitation case load, and the specific functions the rehabilitation team wishes to assess and monitor.

Besides the floor and ceiling effects, the rehabilitation team must consider the functional assessment scale in terms of:

- Validity (the extent to which a test measures what it is supposed to measure):
  - Content validity
  - Face validity
  - Predictive validity
  - Concurrent validity
  - Construct validity
- Reliability (the degree to which a test consistently measures whatever it measures and expressed in terms of standard error of measurement):
  - Test-retest reliability
  - Alternate-forms reliability
  - Split-half reliability
  - Rationale equivalence reliability
  - Internal consistency reliability

Table 2. Examples of commonly used functional measurement tools.

1. Measurements for impairments
Spinal cord injury: American Spinal Injury Association (ASIA) Impairment Scale
Stroke: Fugl-Meyer Scales of Upper Limb and Lower Limb; Trunk Impairment Scale
Traumatic brain injury: Ranchos Los Amigos Cognitive Scale; Westmead Post-Traumatic Amnesia Score
Musculoskeletal: Manual Muscle Testing
Neurological: Modified Ashworth Scale for Spasticity (MAS)
Cognition: Montreal Cognitive Assessment (MoCA)
2. Measurements for activity limitations

a. Activities of Daily Living (ADL) Scales:
  i. Modified Barthel Index (MBI)
  ii. Functional Independence Measure (FIM)
  iii. Modified Functional Ambulation Classifications (MFAC)
  iv. Timed Up and Go Test (TUG)

b. Scales for specific impairments of body structures or body parts:
  i. Lower Limb Amputation: Amputee Mobility Predictor Instrument (AMPI); Medicare K Classification of Prosthetic Use
  ii. Traumatic Brain Injury: Disability Rating Scale (DRS); Functional Assessment Measures (FAM)

3. Measurements for participation restrictions

a. Quality of Life Scales: Short Form-36 (SF36), Euro-Quality-of-Life-5 Dimensions (EQ-5D)

b. Extended ADL Scales: Instrumental ADL

Not everything that can be counted counts
and not everything that counts can be counted.

Albert Einstein

2

Deconditioning and Immobility in Hospitalised Patients

TAN Ping Ping

Definition of deconditioning

- "To lose fitness" or reduced physiological adaptation to normal conditions.

- It is a complex process of physiological changes following a period of inactivity, bedrest or sedentary lifestyle.

- Deconditioning results in functional losses in the areas of mental status, degree of continence and ability to manage self care.

Degree of deconditioning

- Mild: difficulty with maximal activity

- Moderate: difficulty with normal activity

- Severe: difficulty with minimal activity and self care

Pathophysiology of deconditioning

Cardiovascular changes

- Increase in resting heart rate (4–15 beats per minute within first 3–4 weeks, then plateaus)

- Fluid shifts and decrease in blood volume (5% in 24 hours, 10% in 1 week, 20% in 2 weeks)

- Orthostatic (postural) hypotension

- Relative pro-thrombotic state (increased risk of deep venous thrombosis and pulmonary embolism)

- Bed rest → 500–700 ml of fluid from the lower extremities to shift to the thorax → increased stroke volume/cardiac output/left end-diastolic volume

- Relative increase in blood volume in the chest → increased "stretch" in the baroreceptors, and a decrease in heart rate and contractility, vasodilatation, venodilatation and diuresis
- However with prolonged bedrest → decreased levels of aldosterone and anti-diuretic hormone → diuresis (with decreased blood and plasma volume) → increased heart rate and stroke volume to maintain cardiac output → increased orthostatic hypotension

Respiratory changes

- Immediate decrease in all pulmonary function parameters (related to fluid shift and the diaphragm moving to a more cephalad position) → overall reduced muscle strength and endurance → reduced movements of the diaphragmatic, intercostal and abdominal muscles → pooling of mucus and impaired ciliary functions in the airways → impaired cough → mucus plugging and atelectasis→ increased risk of respiratory infections

Musculoskeletal changes

1. Muscle weakness

- Secondary to disuse → atrophy
- Main structural changes include a decrease in diameter and size of muscle fibres, reduced compliance to stretch, reduced number of sarcomeres in series and peak tetanic tension, relative increase in connective tissue, weakness and reduction of endurance and fitness
- With total inactivity, there will be a 10–20% decrease in muscle strength per week (approximately 1–3 % per day)
- Greatest loss will be experienced in the anti-gravity/postural muscles (quadriceps and gastrocnemius-soleus muscle groups)
- Muscle fibres and connective tissues are maintained in a shortened position (5–7 days)
- Muscle fibres and connective tissues adapt to shortened position by contraction of collagen fibres and decrease in muscle fibre sarcomeres
- Loose connective tissues in muscles and around the joint gradually change into dense connective tissue (in approximately 3 weeks)
- Increased risk of compression/entrapment neuropathy (especially in peroneal and ulnar nerves)

2. Disuse osteoporosis

- Loss of bone density due to increased bone resorption secondary to lack of weight bearing, gravity and muscle activity on bone mass, especially in the long bones.

3. Joint changes

- Joint contractures (hips, knees, ankles, shoulders)
- Synovial atrophy
- Cartilage degeneration
- Fibrofatty connective tissue infiltration

Skin changes

- Dependent edema
- Increased risk of pressure ulceration (extrinsic pressure > than capillary perfusion pressure of 30 mmHg for prolonged time) → increased risk of ischemia to affected tissue

Gastrointestinal, nutritional and metabolic changes

- Decreased appetite
- Decreased gastric secretion
- Atrophy of intestinal mucosa and glands
- Constipation
- Slower rate of absorption
- Altered taste
- Decreased lean body mass
- Increased body fat
- Altered nitrogen balance, loss of mineral and electrolyes
- Impaired glucose tolerance
- Altered circadian rhythm
- Altered temperature and sweating response

- Altered regulation of hormones (parathyroid, thyroid, adrenal, pituitary, growth, androgens, and plasma renin activity)

Urological changes

- Increased diuresis and mineral excretion → increased risk of stone formation (especially in association with incomplete bladder emptying) → increased risk of urinary tract infection

Neurocognitive and psychological changes

- Adverse psycho-physiological responses during partial confinement in bed and accompanying hospital routine (changes in the physical environment, restricted food/fluid intake, constipation, altered taste sensitivity)

- Reduced visual acuity, hearing

- Lack of social stimulation can lead to changes in affect (anxiety, fear, neurosis, depression), cognition (reduced concentration, impaired judgment and problem solving), perception (disorientation to time/space, hallucinations, reduced pain threshold, increased auditory threshold) and behaviour (increased risk of psychosis, increased apathy, increased irritability, decreased participation)

Differential diagnosis (especially in critical care areas or in post critical care patients)

- Physical deconditioning

- Intensive care unit-associated weakness

- Critical illness myopathy/polyneuropathy/mixed

- Secondary postural tachycardia syndrome

Interventions that are useful

- Early mobilisation (e.g. sit up in bed, sit over edge of bed, sit to stand, march on the spot, sit out of bed), timely referral to the physiotherapist/occupational therapist

- Frequent changes in position/pressure relief, skin care

- Maintaining functional position of head, trunk, arms, hands, legs and feet
- Deep breathing, coughing and incentive spirometry
- Adequate hydration and nutrition
- Active or passive range of motion exercises with terminal stretches, progressive stretching
- Maintenance of continence, timed void schedule, void on commode/upright whenever appropriate
- Maintenance of a normal sleep-wake cycle
- Visual aids, hearing aids, dentures availability whenever appropriate
- Music, photos, books whenever appropriate
- Progressive tilt table conditioning, standing frame
- Ambulation (assisted)
- Exercise program: endurance, coordination/balance, flexibility, strengthening/resistive
- Combination of progressive resistive exercises for strength and flexibility to antigravity muscles and functional training in mobility can prevent and treat muscle atrophy

3
Stroke Rehabilitation

RATHA KRISHNA Rathi, YAP Giok Mei Samantha

Introduction

Stroke is the fourth leading cause of death and the leading cause of disability in Singapore. With an aging population, its prevalence is likely to increase. Stroke rehabilitation aims to improve functional outcomes following stroke, therefore reducing the burden of care on society, caregivers and improving the independence and dignity of the patient.

Common stroke deficits

- Motor
    - At the onset of hemiplegia, arm is often more involved than the leg. Motor recovery in the leg occurs earlier and is more complete than in the arm
- Sensory impairment
- Cognitive disorders
    - Most powerful negative factor for outcome
    - Most common are impairments in attention, memory and executive functioning
- Visual perceptual disorders
    - Manifest as apraxia, agnosia, hemi-neglect, homonymous hemianopia
- Dysphasia
- Dysphagia
- Bowel/bladder dysfunction
- Emotional disturbance

Common terminology used to describe stroke deficits

1. Hemiplegic gait:

    (a) Asymmetric gait pattern with decreased gait speed, increased stance time on unaffected limb

    (b) Loss of normal reciprocal arm motion of gait on affected arm which may be flaccid initially in the early stages or positioned in adduction and flexion in the later stages

    (c) Affected lower limb shows extensor synergy pattern (extension, adduction, internal rotation of hip; extension of knee; plantarflexion/inversion foot/ankle)

    (d) Due to extended limb posture causing difficulty with adequate limb clearance during swing phase, there may be associated compensatory manoeuvres including hip hiking, lateral trunk sway, circumduction and less commonly, contralateral vaulting

2. Apraxia: disorder of voluntary movement where one cannot execute a purposeful activity despite the presence of adequate mobility, strength, sensation, coordination and comprehension

    (a) Apraxia of speech: highly variable and unpredictable substitutions of sounds

    (b) Ideomotor apraxia: inability to automatically perform a movement and unable to repeat it on command (e.g. unable to walk on command)

    (c) Ideational apraxia: inability to coordinate individual steps into an integrated sequence (e.g. holds toothbrush but does not bring it to the mouth)

3. Agnosia: disorder of recognition that may occur in any of the major sense modalities despite adequate perception in these modalities:

    (a) Auditory agnosia: unable to match environmental noise with sound source

    (b) Visual agnosia: unable to identify object on visual confrontation

    (c) Anosognosia: unaware of loss of an important bodily function, primarily hemiplegia

4. Hemi-neglect: disorder of attention with failure to report, respond, or orient to sensory stimuli presented to the side contralateral to the stroke. In severe neglect, patients often collide with objects on the affected side, ignoring

objects in front of them and attending to only one side of the body. In milder forms of neglect, patients present with various degrees of ignoring the affected side when faced with stimulation on the affected side

5. Homonymous hemianopia: visual field defect involving either the two right or the two left halves of the visual fields of both eyes. It is caused by lesions of the retrochiasmal visual pathways often involving the occipital lobe

6. Dysphagia: defined as difficulty swallowing and may be divided into oropharyngeal or oesophageal dysphagia. Common terminology often used in dysphagia includes:

    (a) Laryngeal penetration: entrance of food in the airway to the level of the true vocal folds

    (b) Aspiration: passage of food below the level of the true vocal folds

    (c) Silent aspiration: absence of any outward signs of difficulty during swallowing

7. Dysarthria: impairment in articulation of words. May be flaccid, spastic or ataxic

8. Aphasia: a language disorder characterised by impaired communication

Table 1. Aphasia classification.

	Fluency	Comprehension	Repetition	Lesion
Global	Poor	Poor	Poor	MCA (middle cerebral artery), multilobes
Transcortical mixed	Poor	Poor	Good	ACA (anterior cerebral artery)/PCA (posterior cerebral artery), watershed areas
Broca's	Poor	Good	Poor	MCA, frontal
Transcortical motor	Poor	Good	Good	ACA, prefrontal
Wernicke's	Good	Poor	Poor	MCA, temporal
Transcortical sensory	Good	Poor	Good	PCA, parietooccipital
Conduction	Good	Good	Poor	MCA, arcuate fasciculus

    (a) Other types of aphasia include:

    ■ Alexia: inability to recognize or read written words or letters

    ■ Anomia: poor naming

Stroke recovery

Mechanism of stroke recovery

- Neurological recovery
    - Recovery of impairments due to
        - Resolution of oedema (up to 8 weeks)
        - Reperfusion of ischaemic penumbra
        - Resolution of diaschisis
        - Neuroplasticity (cortical reorganisation)
- Functional recovery
    - Improvement in activities of daily living and mobility due to recovery of impairment and/or compensation/adaptation
    - Can continue to improve for sometime after neurological recovery is complete

Time course to recovery

- Peak neurological recovery occurs within first 1–3 months
- Recovery continues at a slower pace up to 6 months
- Up to 5% continue to recover up to 1 year
- Progress toward recovery may plateau at any stage of recovery
- ~10% moderate to severe stroke achieve "full" recovery
- Depends on the initial severity of impairments

N.B. Return of motor power is NOT recovery of function. Function may be impaired by other deficits associated with stroke such as cognitive impairments, in-coordination, apraxias, sensory and communication problems.

Prognostic factors in stroke

- Age > 74 years
- Prolonged flaccidity of paralysed limb
- Right hemisphere lesion with hemi-neglect

- Cognitive impairment
- Anterior circulation
- Large lesion size
- Severity of stroke (determines capacity for neuroplasticity, inverse relationship between stroke size and recovery)

Factors affecting outcome in stroke

- Intensity of therapy ("more is better" resulting in improved overall functional outcomes and shorter hospital stay)
- Stroke rehabilitation unit
- Early rehabilitation (results in greater brain plasticity hence better outcomes)
- Family support

Motor function recovery following stroke

Brunnstrom stages of motor recovery (describes the evolution of hemiplegia)

I. Flaccidity

II. Some spasticity, basic synergy patterns, minimal movements may be present

III. Increase in spasticity, some voluntary control over synergies

IV. Decrease in spasticity, some selective activation of muscles outside synergy pattern

V. Further decrease in spasticity, most limb movements outside synergy pattern

VI. Disappearance of spasticity, near normal coordination with isolated movements

VII. Normal function restored

Depending on stroke severity and recovery potential, the stages may progress quickly or may be skipped. Generally, hemiplegia with short or absent stage I has better recovery i.e. the longer the stage I, the worse the prognosis; the lower the stage, the poorer the outcome.

Poor prognostic indicators for upper limb (UL) recovery

- Severe proximal spasticity
- No propioceptive facilitation response > 9 days
- No onset of movement at > 2–4 weeks
- Absence of voluntary hand movement at 4–6 weeks
- Prolonged flaccid period

Poor prognostic indicators for independent walking

- Poor sitting balance
- Poor truncal control
- Urinary incontinence
- Severity of disability
- Age > 74 years

Types of motor rehabilitation therapies post stroke

- **Neurodevelopemental technique (Bobath approach)**
  - Goal is to normalise tone, inhibit primitive patterns of movement, and facilitate automatic, voluntary reactions and subsequent normal movement patterns
  - Most commonly used approach
  - Opposite of Brunnstrom approach
- **Brunnstrom method**
  - Uses primitive postural reactions and synergies to facilitate motor function
  - Encourages the use of abnormal movement
  - Opposite of Neurodevelopmental technique
- **Propioceptive neuromuscular facilitation (PNF)**
  - Uses spiral, diagonal techniques to facilitate movements

- **Rood method (sensorimotor approach)**
  - Uses cutaneous sensorimotor stimuli to activate motor function and inhibit spastic antagonists (e.g. icing, brushing, vibration)
- **Motor relearning program (Carr and Shepard approach)**
  - Relearn how to move functionally and how to problem solve during attempts at new tasks
  - Emphasises task-specific functional training

Other therapeutic approaches to stroke rehabilitation
Constraint-induced movement therapy (CIMT)

- Forced use of the paralysed arm to promote cortical reorganisation of the brain which in turn leads to recovery of upper limb function
- Benefit patients with no significant spasticity and who have some strength of the paralysed upper extremity, especially those with sensory loss and neglect
- Involves
  - (a) Participation in an intensive upper extremity therapy program for 6 hours per day, using the affected limb during the same 2-week period
  - (b) Restriction of less affected upper limb up to 90% of waking hours during 2-week period
  - (c) Shaping therapy, a training method in which a motor task is gradually made more difficult as patient gains skills
- Criteria for CIMT
  - Higher-functioning participants
    - At least 20° of wrist extension and at least 10° of active extension of each metacarpophalangeal and interphalangeal joint of all digits
  - Lower-functioning participants
    - At least 10° of active wrist extension, at least 10° of thumb abduction/extension, and at least 10° of extension in at least 2 additional digits

Task-specific training

- Train specifically for a given task

- Involves repetition and skilled motor relearning
- Yields longer lasting cortical reorganisation specific to the corresponding areas being used
- Mobility task-specific training is associated with improvements in walking distance, speed and balance
- Allows for best recovery

Body weight-supported treadmill training (BWSTT)

- Locomotor retraining on treadmill with partial body weight support
- Enables repetitive practice of complex gait cycles rather than single limb preparatory manoeuvres
- Goal is for symmetrical gait, less spasticity, better gait speed and energy conservation
- Combination of task-specific and strength training
- Criteria for treadmill training with body weight support
    - Able to understand simple instructions
    - Able to stand with or without support for at least 30 min
    - No osteoporosis
    - No acute lower limb fractures or severe pain

Functional electrical stimulation (FES)

- Uses electrical current to generate muscle contraction, hence movement
- Used to improve strength, spasticity, range of motion and function
- Used in lower limb foot drop, upper limb wrist drop, shoulder pain and subluxation

Rehabilitation of stroke deficits
Rehabilitation of neglect

- Tests used for screening of neglect
    - Line bisection
    - Single letter cancellation

- Behavioural inattention test

Interventions for management of neglect include:

- Increasing patient's awareness of or attention to the neglected space
  - Visual scanning: consistently scan to involved side
  - Arousal strategies: using external sensory stimulus
  - Activation strategies: i.e. spatial motor cueing (limb activation and/or application of sensory stimulation)
  - Feedback to increase awareness of neglect behaviour involving auditory and visual stimuli
- Compensatory technique focusing on targeting deficits with a specific intervention
  - Use of prisms: optical deviation of visual fields to affected side
  - Eye patching: increase eye movements to contralateral space
  - Hemispatial glasses
  - Transcutaneous electrical nerve stimulation (TENS): a form of sensory stimulation

Rehabilitation of dysphasia

- Tests used to screen for dysphasia include:
  - Frenchay aphasia screening test
  - Porch index of communicative ability
- Interventions for dysphasia include:
  - Behavioural approach
    - Intensive speech and language therapy
    - Melodic intonation therapy
    - Constraint induced aphasia therapy
  - Biologic approach
    - Neuropharmacology (e.g. piracetam , L-dopa, amphetamine, donezepil, memantine)
    - Transcranial magnetic or electrical stimulation (fostering brain neuroplasticity)

- Alternative augmentative communication
  - Use of writing, drawing, communication books, electronic communication devices

Rehabilitation of dysphagia after stroke

- Screening and assessment of dysphagia after stroke include:
  - Bedside clinical test with 3oz water swallow test
  - Instrumental assessment
    - Videofluroscopy (VFS)/modified barium swallow (gold standard)
      - Advantages:
        - √ Able to assess impairment at each stage of swallowing,
        - √ Able to describe mechanism of laryngeal penetration/aspiration
        - √ Able to directly visualise the effects of compensatory strategies to facilitate safe and effective swallowing
      - Disadvantages:
        - √ Exposure to small amounts of radiation
        - √ Food is coated with barium hence taste may be altered
        - √ Test cannot be done in patients who cannot sit upright in a chair
    - Flexible endoscopic evaluation of swallowing (FEES)
      - Advantages:
        - √ Allows direct viewing of larynx
        - √ Food is laced with coloured dye, no contrast needed, taste of food not changed.
        - √ Can be used in "practice swallows" to determine safest patient position and food texture
        - √ Can be done at the bedside
        - √ Investigates both motor and sensory components of swallowing
      - Disadvantages:
        - √ May experience mild discomfort, gagging, vomiting, vasovagal syncope, epistaxis

√ Risk of laryngospasm and inhalation of the bolus

√ Only investigates pharyngeal stage of swallowing

√ No visualisation of the actual swallow because of "whiteout", hence details of oral and pharyngeal motility must be inferred

- Interventions for dysphagia include:
    - Modification of diet: thickened fluids or modified food textures
    - Enteral feeding for those who are unable to swallow
    - Swallow using swallowing compensatory manoeuvres such as:
        - Mendelsohn manoeuvre: patient holds the larynx up, either using the muscles of the neck or with the hand, during the swallow, for an extended period of time increasing airway protection
        - Masako manoeuvre: patient protrudes tongue to increase pharyngeal constriction and then swallows
        - Chin tuck: patient flexes the neck before swallow to prevent premature spillage over base of tongue; increasing airway protection by widening the vallecula and putting the epiglottis in a more overhanging position
        - Supraglottic swallow: patient takes a deep breath, holds it and swallows. This adducts the vocal folds and increases the strength of swallowing muscles thus improving airway protection
        - Effortful swallow: patient squeezes all the muscles of swallowing as hard as he can and then swallows
        - Head/neck rotation: patient turns the head/neck to the weaker side, closing off that side and swallows. This directs the food to the stronger side
- Swallowing exercises to improve strength of swallowing muscles
    - Shaker exercise: lifting and maintaining head in flexed position while lying flat
    - Thermal/tactile stimulation of oropharynx: improves initiation and timing of swallow response
    - Oro-motor exercises to improve oral manipulation and control of boluses

- Mendelsohn manoeuvre: see above. Exercise done without food
    - Supraglottic swallow: see above. Exercise done without food
- Alternative interventions for swallowing include neuromuscular electrical stimulation, transcranial direct current stimulation and repetitive transcranial magnetic stimulation

Neuropharmacology in stroke

- Neuropharmacology is often used in post-stroke patients to enhance recovery.
- Motor recovery
    - Selective serotonin receptor inhibitors (SSRIs) have been found to alter motor recovery by modulating neuronal plasticity. The use of SSRIs has been found to be associated with improvement in neurological impairment, disability and dependence
    - Medications commonly used include fluoxetine and citalopram
- Cognitive impairment
    - Up to 39% of patients have cognitive impairments at one year post-stroke. The presence of cognitive deficits affects functional ability and is also associated with depression
    - Medications used include:
        - Cholinesterase inhibitors (e.g. donepezil, galantamine, rivastigmine)
        - Memantine (NMDA receptor antagonist)
        - Methylphenidate: 10–15 mg/day up to 60 mg/day in 2–3 divided doses
- Post-stroke depression
    - Post-stroke depression affects 23–40% of stroke patients. Pharmacologic treatment of depression is associated with improved functional recovery post stroke and improved long term survival
    - Medications used include:
        - Heterocyclic antidepressants (e.g. amitriptyline, nortriptyline)
        - Selective serotonin reuptake inhibitors (e.g. fluoxetine, sertraline, citalopram)

- Psychostimulants (e.g. methylphenidate)

- Aphasia

  - Neuropharmacologic treatment has been associated with aphasia recovery

  - Medications used in aphasia therapy include piracetam, L-dopa, amphetamine and donezepil

Scales used in rehabilitation

Specific neurologic impairment scales (to measure specific types of deficits)

- Motor impairments

  - Fugl-Meyer assessment

  - Motor assessment scale

  - Motricity index

- Balance

  - Berg balance scale

  - Trunk control test

- Arm/hand function

  - Action research arm test

- Mobility

  - Rivermead mobility index

- Aphasia

  - Frenchay aphasia screening test

  - Porch index of communicative ability

- Cognition

  - Montreal cognitive assessment (MoCA)

Disability scales

- Barthel index (BI)
  - 10 basic aspects of self-care and physical dependency
  - Floor and ceiling effects
  - Insensitive to change in function at the extreme ends of the scale

Table 2. Barthel index.

Barthel Index	Level of dependency
100	Nil (normal)
> 60	Assisted independence
40–60	Moderate dependency
< 40	Severe dependency

- Functional independence measure (FIM)
  - 13 aspects of motor function, 5 aspects of cognitive function
  - Monitors functional improvement through the course of rehabilitation therapy

Handicap scales

- Modified Rankin scale
  - Measures functional independence on a 7 grade scale
  - Measure of stroke-related handicap
  - Global measure of the functional impact of stroke

Table 3. Modified Rankin scale.

Score	Description
0	No symptoms at all
1	No significant disability despite symptoms; able to carry out all usual duties and activities
2	Slight disability; unable to carry out all previous activities, but able to look after own affairs without assistance
3	Moderate disability; requiring some help, but able to walk without assistance
4	Moderately severe disability; unable to walk without assistance and unable to attend to own bodily needs without assistance
5	Severe disability; bedridden, incontinent and requiring constant nursing care and attention
6	Dead

Emerging rehabilitation modalities

- Non-invasive brain stimulation

- Transcranial direct current stimulation (tDCS)

- Repetitive transcranial magnetic stimulation (rTMS)

- Brain-computer interface facilitated therapy

- Biotherapeutics

Blood markers associated with stroke risk

- Role of blood biomarkers in stroke is limited

- Several are associated with stroke outcomes namely

  - Brain natriuretic peptide (BNP)

  - C- Reactive Protein (CRP)

  - Fibrinogen

  - Lipoprotein- associated phospholipase A2 (LP-PLA2)

  - S100 calcium binding protein B

4
Spinal Cord Injury Rehabilitation

TAN En-Xian Emily, WONG Chin Jung, TOW Peh Er Adela

Causes of spinal cord injury (SCI)

(a) Traumatic: road traffic accident, falls, assault.

(b) Non-traumatic: cervical spondylotic myelopathy, prolapsed intervertebral disc, rheumatoid arthritis, spinal tumours (metastatic > primary), spinal cord infarction, spinal cord vascular malformation, spine infections (epidural abscess, spondylodiscitis), transverse myelitis

Assessment of SCI patient on admission to rehabilitation

(a) Review premorbid function, history of injury or illness, surgical/ medical interventions

(b) Check baseline blood pressure (BP) and orthostatic hypotension, weight bearing or range of motion (ROM) restrictions, pressure ulcers (especially sacrum and heel), sitting tolerance, cognition and psychological status

(c) Medication review: analgesia, deep vein thrombosis (DVT) prophylaxis, sedatives, laxatives

(d) Bowel and bladder charting, intake and output chart. Exclude dysphagia if anterior cervical fixation done—refer to speech therapist

International Standards for Neurological Classification of SCI (ISNCSCI)

- References for the 2011 revision of the international standards for neurological classification of spinal cord injury:

  - http://www.ncbi.nlm.nih.gov/pmc/articles/PMC3232637/

- http://www.iscos.org.uk/sitefiles/PageFile_20_Motor_Exam_Guide.pdf
- http://www.iscos.org.uk/sitefiles/PageFile_20_Key_Sensory_Points.pdf

Pinprick sensation (sharp/dull discrimination)

- Both light touch and pin prick to be tested in respective dermatomes
- Note for normal examination requires both sharp/dull discrimination and sensation of sharpness to be same as that on the face
- Lowest normal level for all modalities taken as sensory level on that side

Motor examination and level

- Note motor examination requires full ROM against gravity for grade 3, full ROM gravity eliminated for grade 2
- Motor level—the most caudal key muscle with a grade of 3 and above, provided the key muscles above it are graded 5
- Reason: each designated muscle has 2 root innervations, if power of 3/5 = full innervation by more rostral root level
- For myotomes not clinically testable, i.e. C1 to C4, T2 to L1, and S2 to S5, motor level is same as sensory level if motor function above is normal
- Right and left, sensory and motor levels are determined separately
- Neurological level of injury (NLI)—most rostral of the normal sensory and right and left motor levels

Asia Impairment Scale (AIS): A to E

- Complete: (AIS A) absent sensory or motor function in the most sacral segment (S4/5) including absent voluntary anal sphincter and anal sensation
- Incomplete (AIS B, C D, E): preserved light touch, pinprick, deep anal sensation at S4-5 or voluntary anal contraction present
- Worksheet: http://asia-spinalinjury.org/wp-content/uploads/2016/02/International_Stds_Diagram_Worksheet.pdf
- Online algorithms: http://www.isncscialgorithm.com

SCI clinical syndromes

- Central cord syndrome: hyperextension injury from fall; background spondylosis; upper limbs more affected than lower limbs

- Brown Sequard syndrome: ipsilateral motor and proprioception loss; contralateral loss of pain and temperature; usually good prognosis

- Anterior cord syndrome: anterior spinal artery injury; flaccid paralysis; prognosis is poorer if there is spinothalamic function impairment—loss of motor and pinprick

- Posterior cord syndrome: dorsal column injury; loss of proprioception and vibration

- Cauda equina syndrome: flaccid paralysis and sensory impairment of the lower limbs depending on nerve roots involved +/- areflexic bowel and bladder. Sacral reflexes, i.e. bulbocavernosus and anal wink will be absent

- Conus medullaris: terminal segment of the adult spinal cord; mixed picture of reflexic (due to conus injury) and areflexic signs (due to nerve root injury)

Common cardiovascular complications
Autonomic dysreflexia

- This is a medical emergency. If left untreated, the rise in BP can result in cerebral hemorrhage, myocardial infarction and seizures. Prompt recognition and management is essential

- Massive sympathetic discharge in lesions at T6 and above; usually seen in complete injuries

- Sudden rise in BP > 20–40 mmHg above baseline with noxious stimulus

- Tachycardia/bradycardia, headache, perspiration; flushing, piloerection, pupillary constriction, sinus congestion; cardiac arrhythmias: seizures, intracranial haemorrhage, myocardial infarction

- Noxious stimulus below level of injury stimulates sympathetic system → splanchnic vasoconstriction → rise in BP; carotid baroreceptors cause reflex bradycardia, vasodilation above the level of lesion

- Management
    - Aim to reduce BP and remove inciting stimulus
    - Sit patient upright, elevate head

- Loosen all tight fitting clothing and devices
- Flush indwelling catheter (IDC) if blocked. Change IDC—need to use local anaesthetic, e.g. lignocaine gel when inserting IDC
- Monitor BP and pulse every 2–5 minutes during episode
  - Exclude and check for inciting stimuli and treat accordingly
    - √ Bladder: retention of urine, blocked catheter, urinary tract infection
    - √ Faecal impaction; pressure ulcers, ingrown toenails, tight clothing
    - √ Abdominal causes: appendicitis, cholecystitis, gastric ulcers
    - √ Other causes: bladder stone, limb fractures
    - √ Females: menstrual cramps, during labour/delivery
- If BP does not decrease despite physical measures, consider using medications: sublingual nifedipine 5 mg or sublingual captopril 25 mg; monitor BP until it returns to patient's normal

Orthostatic hypotension

- Poor venous return; loss of sympathetically mediated reflex vasoconstriction when tilted > 60 degrees; peripheral pooling of blood; cardiovascular deconditioning
- Management
  - Avoid quick upright positioning
  - Review anti-hypertensives, alpha-blockers for benign prostatic hyperplasia, etc.
  - Compression stockings, abdominal binder; progressive sitting program
  - Adequate salt and water intake
  - Medications—fludrocortisone, midodrine

Thrombo-prophylaxis in SCI patients

- Hypercoagulability, stasis and intimal injury (Virchow's triad)
- Management

- Mechanical prophylaxis in all—anti-thromboembolic stockings, e.g. TEDS +/- external pneumatic devices/foot pumps

- Complete injury—subcutaneous clexane for 8 (uncomplicated) to 12 weeks (other risk factors, e.g. lower limb fractures, heart failure, cancer, age > 70 years)

- Incomplete injury—anticoagulants continued until discharge

- Suspected pulmonary embolism: venous ultrasound, venography, D-dimer, CT pulmonary angiogram

Respiratory issues and management

Anatomy and pathophysiology

- Inspiratory muscles: diaphragm, external intercostals, accessory muscles

- Expiratory muscles: abdominal muscles, internal intercostals

- Innervation: diaphragm: phrenic nerve (C3, 4, 5)

Post-SCI

- Tetraplegics and high paraplegics: erect posture — diaphragm biomechanically disadvantaged

- Decreased vital capacity (VC) and tidal volume (TV)

- Secretions, bronchospasm; reduction in chest wall compliance

- Pneumonia, atelectasis, and respiratory failure are commoner in high tetraplegics

- Dyspnoea, paradoxical breathing — poor chest expansion

Management

- Prevent complications, restore pulmonary function to the highest possible level by maximising breathing capacity and enhancing cough ability

- Maximal inspiratory/expiratory chest X-ray — exclude diaphragmatic paralysis

- Lung function test — forced vital capacity (FVC), peak cough flow (PCF)

Maximise breathing capacity

- Abdominal binder when upright — stabilise lower rib cage; improve diaphragmatic efficiency

- Deep breathing exercises +/- incentive spirometry — deep breath, holding and taking, repeating a few breaths before slowly breathing out; adding incentive spirometry provides visual feedback

- Inspiratory muscle training (IMT) — devices that increase the resistive or threshold inspiratory load for improving strength

- Glossopharyngeal breathing (GPB) — "frog breathing" to augment vital capacity; muscles of the mouth and pharynx used to propel small volumes of air through larynx; glottis is used to trap air into lungs

- Breath stacking with bag valve mask — lung volume recruitment (LVR) after breathing in maximally, augmented breath increases lung volume over and above vital capacity

- Contraindications — haemoptysis, pneumothorax, bullous emphysema, nausea, severe chronic obstructive airways disease or asthma and recent lobectomy, increased intra-cranial pressure, ventricular drains

Secretion management and enhancing cough abilities

- Effective cough — requires large inspiratory volume and an expulsive expiration. All complete tetraplegics require manually assisted cough as the intercostals and abdominal strength needed to generate cough are absent

- Measure PCF

  - PCF < 270 L/min is associated with poor cough and high risk of respiratory infection; requires manual cough assist and also LVR (via breath stacking with bag valve mask)

  - PCF < 160 L/min — despite LVR and manual cough assist — additionally requires mechanical cough assist with mechanical insufflation-exsufflation (MIE)

  - Manual cough assist — increases peak expiratory flow rate (PEFR) during cough — using modified Heimlich manoeuvre — assists cough by timing with patient's expiration; contraindications — presence of inferior vena cava (IVC) filters, acute abdominal or chest injuries

- MIE device (cough assist device) — provides deep inspiration (positive pressure) followed rapidly by controlled suction (negative pressure); rapid pressure change induces a high expiratory flow similar to a cough; less traumatic than suctioning; usually done 1 — 3 times daily. Precaution— watch for pneumothorax or pneumo-mediastinum

Tracheostomy weaning

- Criteria for readiness of decannulation:
  - Vital signs stable — afebrile for 3 days; clear chest X-ray (CXR); no aspiration; minimal secretions, suctioning requirements less than 3 times a day; oxygen saturation > 92% room air; effective quad cough/manually assisted cough
  - Uncuff cuffed tubes, change to cuffless tube; decrease cannula diameter; speaking valve — option of phonation; increase tolerance for capping
  - Ear, nose and throat (ENT) referral — exclude tracheal/glottic stenosis; tracheal granuloma
  - Tendency to fatigue — spigotting in multiple short trials progressively; start with 5–10 mins daily → 10–15 mins bd → 30 mins bd, and progress according to tolerance; when tolerating > 24 hrs with no desaturation, good cough and minimal secretions, patient is ready for decannulation

Sleep disordered breathing

- More common in complete tetraplegics than normal population
- Obstructive sleep apnoea (OSA), central sleep apnoea, sleep related hypoventilation
- Symptoms — daytime sleepiness, unrefreshed sleep, fatigue
- Overnight oximetry/portable sleep devices → full polysomnography if positive
- Management
  - Sleeping in lateral rather than supine; weight loss
  - Non-invasive ventilation: auto continuous positive airway pressure (CPAP) in OSA, CPAP and back up rate in central sleep apnoea, bilevel positive airway pressure (BIPAP) and back up rate for sleep related hypoventilation

Bladder management

- Disruption in the spinal cord between sacral nerves and the pontine micturition centre → inability to coordinate detrusor and sphincter for voiding and storage

- **Overactive bladder** → overactive sacral reflexes +/- detrusor sphincter dyssynergia (DSD)

- **Underactive bladder** → flaccid bladder, with loss of sacral reflexes

Investigations

- Bladder diary: intake of fluids, voiding frequency, voided volumes, nocturnal voiding, urgency, incontinence episodes and residual urine

- Baseline upper tract evaluation: ultrasound (US) kidneys and bladder

- Post-void residual (PVR) should be done in patients who are able to void

Aims of bladder management

- Preservation of upper tract function, improvement of urinary continence, restoration of lower urinary tract function, improve quality of life

Management scenarios

Scenario 1: patient admitted on IDC

- Keep IDC until medical complications resolved,

- Trial off catheter when medically stable, absence of urinary tract infection (UTI), urinary output is < 2 L/day

- Trial of voiding (remove IDC)

    - Typically done early in the morning

    - Complete tetraplegics — observe for AD symptoms with bladder filling

    - Monitor BP and heart rate half hourly; if patient has autonomic dysreflexia, abandon trial

- If patient is unable to void with catheter off, do intermittent catheterisation hourly and note incontinent episodes in between

Scenario 2: patient able to void spontaneously

- Note if urge or incontinence is present
- Check post void residual volume (PVR) and do clean intermittent catheterisation if PVR > 150–200 ml

Scenario 3: patient admitted on collecting device (diapers)

- Trial of off diapers: 3–4 hourly potting and check PVR

Urodynamic studies (UDS)

- To classify the neurogenic bladder dysfunction
- Predict which patients will develop complications and require early intervention
- Identify factors contributing to incontinence for management

Before UDS

- Exclude urinary tract infection; clear bowels one day before
- Discontinue drugs that influence bladder function or note medication use during interpretation

UDS parameters

- Storage phase
  - Detrusor: normal/overactive
  - Compliance: low/normal
  - Cystometric capacity: normal/low
  - Detrusor leak point pressure
  - Sensation: reduced, normal
- Voiding phase
  - Detrusor: normal/hypocontractile/acontractile
  - Maximal detrusor pressure
  - Urethral/outflow function: detrusor sphincter dyssynergia (DSD); outflow obstruction
  - PVR

- Urinary incontinence/storage failure may result from detrusor overactivity, atonic detrusor with overflow (high volumes) and pelvic floor insufficiency
- Urinary retention/voiding failure may result from underactive/hypocontractile detrusor, outlet obstruction (persistent sympathetic tone, DSD; urethral stricture, enlarged prostate)

Management of storage failure

- Neurogenic overactive bladder/low compliance (with or without DSD)
- Normal PVR volume does not mean the presence of a safe bladder
- UDS: high pressure filling phase, low compliance, low bladder capacity
- Bladder pressure > 40 mmHg — risk of hydronephrosis
- Management: conversion of high-pressure bladder into low-pressure reservoir despite the resulting residual urine
  - Medications
    - Anti-muscarinics — oxybutynin, tolterodine, solifenacin, darifenacin
    - Tricyclic antidepressants, quarternary ammonium compound (e.g. trospium chloride); side effects: dry mouth, blurred vision, constipation
    - Beta 3 adrenergic agonist — mirabegron; side effects: hypertension, nasopharyngitis, headache, arthralgia, diarrhoea, abdominal pain
  - Empty bladder via intermittent catheterisation
  - Oral medication failure/excessive side effects, consider intravesical botulinum toxin A injection

Management of voiding failure

Underactive detrusor

- Trial of bethanechol 10 mg po tds to facilitate detrusor contraction; outcome is better when the bladder is partially innervated
- Discourage Crede or Valsalva manoeuvre for bladder emptying—risk of high intravesical pressures and vesicoureteral reflux

Outlet obstruction

- Medications

    - Alpha adrenergic antagonist (phenoxybenzamine, terazosin, tamsulosin)

    - Spasmolytic agents (baclofen, diazepam; botulinum toxin injection)

- Sphincterotomy/prostatectomy for BPH; urethrotomy/stent for urethral stricture

Bladder emptying options

Intermittent catheterisation

- Gold standard for management in patients with detrusor underactivity/acontractility and those with detrusor overactivity.

- Frequency: start q4h — adjust frequency/fluid intake; maintain volumes at 400ml

- Clean technique allowed at home — use of soap and tap water to clean hands, no-touch technique. Sterile technique — full aseptic precautions when in hospital

IDC

- Unable to perform intermittent catheterisation or with high urine output

- Temporary management of vesicoureteral reflux/hydronephrosis

- Complications

    - Stones, urethral erosions, epididymitis, recurrent UTI, bladder cancer

- Anticholinergics shown to reduce upper tract complications in chronic IDC

- Consider suprapubic catheterisation for individuals with urethral abnormalities, perineal skin breakdown, body image issues, recurrent prostatitis, urethritis, or epididymo-orchitis

Long term SCI bladder management

- Patients with high pressure bladders — renal US yearly to exclude hydronephrosis

- Serum creatinine or creatinine clearance test yearly

- Cystoscopy every 5–10 years for those on IDC

Bowel management

Aim of bowel program is to achieve consistent and complete clearance of bowels at a specified time, in a timely fashion, with no incontinence, constipation or pain.

Reflex/spastic bowel

- Injury above the conus medullaris — voluntary (cortical) control of stool disrupted, but preserved intrinsic reflexes → incontinence; sphincter tight → retention of stool

- Bowel programme — utilise the gastrocolic and rectocolic reflex (stimulus introduced into the rectum either via suppository or digital stimulation)

- Digital stimulation — gentle insertion and rotation of gloved finger at anus to stimulate rectocolic reflex; repeat every 5–10 min until stool evacuation is complete

- Pharmacological — lactulose; senna ~8 h prior to bowel routine; enema or suppository at the start of the routine

Flaccid/areflexic bowel

- Injury below the conus medullaris — usually L1 and below; areflexic at S2-4 — intrinsic myenteric plexus activity still present

- External anal sphincter and colon both flaccid — increased risk of constipation and incontinence

- Bowel program
    - Add on bulking for easier removal of stool
    - Advised to sit on a commode with the help of Valsalva manouevre
    - Pharmacological measures
        - Dietary fibre > 15 g/day, methylcellulose, psyllium
        - Osmotics — fleet, mannitol, magnesium sulfate
        - Hyperosmotics — PEG, lactulose
        - Stimulants — senna, dulcolax
    - In severely affected individuals, manual removal of the stool may be necessary

Pressure relief measures

- SCI patients are at high risk for pressure ulcers
    - Institute pressure relief measures for all complete SCI
    - 2 hourly turning, pressure relief mattresses frequent pressure relief in wheelchair

Pain

Nociceptive pain

- Musculoskeletal pain (e.g. glenohumeral arthritis, lateral epicondylitis)
- Visceral pain (e.g. myocardial infarction, abdominal pain)
- Other nociceptive pain (e.g. headache, surgical skin incision)

Neuropathic pain

- At level SCI pain (e.g. spinal cord compression, nerve root compression, cauda equina compression)
- Below level SCI pain (e.g. spinal cord ischemia, spinal cord compression)
- Other neuropathic pain (e.g. carpal tunnel syndrome, trigeminal neuralgia)

Shoulder pain in tetraplegics

- Neurological weakness and poor posture → muscle imbalance → anterior tightening; relative weakness of posterior stabilizing muscles
- Chronic impingement, rotator cuff pathology
- Management
    - Proper positioning; back support, improve posture
    - Avoid direct pressure on the shoulder when lying
    - Provide support to the upper limb at all times; when supine, upper limb in abduction and external rotation on a regular basis; avoid pulling on the arm when positioning individuals

Sexuality

Male sexual function in SCI

- Erection: sympathetic T11-L2 (psychogenic); parasympathetic S2-4 (reflex); emission: sympathetic T11- L 2; ejaculation: somatic S2-4

- Erection: in complete lesions above the conus (S2-4), reflex erections (often unpredictable and limited) are preserved; in complete lesions below S2-4, reflex erections are limited and psychogenic erections poorly sustained

- Ejaculation: limited due to interruption of the somatic outflow; commonly, retrograde emission occurs due to inefficient bladder neck closure

Female sexual function in SCI

- Loss of genital sensation and lubrication; changes in arousal and orgasm

Management of erectile dysfunction

- Vacuum erection device

- Oral PDE5 (phosphodiesterase 5) inhibitors: works with sexual arousal → vasodilation; contraindicated with use of nitrates; sildenafil, taladafil (longer half life), vardenafil (avoid in patients with long QT interval)

- Prostaglandin E1, Alprostadil — intracavernosal injection

Fertility issues in females

- Fertility is unaffected; when pregnant, watch for UTI, AD; premature labour may be unrecognised; in lesions above T6, the first / only symptom of labour may be severe AD; epidural anaesthesia gives the best control of AD

Fertility issues in males

- Reproductive capacity may be significantly impaired; referral to fertility centre; semen retrieval can be enhanced using vibro-ejaculation and electro-ejaculation; artificial insemination techniques may be necessary

Will I walk again?

- Generally, most recovery occurs within the first 2 months post-injury, slower rate at 3–6 months, even up to 2 years post-injury. Improvement of at least 1 level adjacent to the last normal level is expected.

- Ambulation potential at 1 year post-injury can be roughly predicted by ASIA Impairment Scale (AIS) assessed within 72 hours post-injury

    - AIS A: 80–90% will remain complete; only 3% recover functional strength in the lower extremities

    - AIS B: overall ambulation ranges from 10–33%

    - AIS C: about 75% will become community ambulators; age and the amount of preserved spinal cord function below the lesion influence recovery of ambulation

    - AIS D: majority will be ambulators

Ambulation training options

- Wheelchair training remains the functional option for those with AIS C and below; strengthening and endurance training of remaining muscles and compensation using braces and assistive devices for support can improve walking in incomplete injuries

- Household ambulation — able to walk in the home; may require assistance with stairs, curbs and ramps outside the home

- Community ambulation — walks outside the home and can manage doors, low curbs and ramps

- Therapeutic ambulation as an option — walking is achieved with maximal assistance and high physiological cost from therapist/caregiver; usually with knee ankle foot orthosis (KAFO)

Functional outcomes by neurological level of injury

Refer to Appendix: Projected functional outcome for tetraplegics

Exercise and activity

- Higher prevalence of cardiovascular disease (30–50%) compared to ambulatory individuals

- Encourage cardiovascular and sports participation early in rehabilitation

- Cardiovascular exercise options: wheelchair wheeling, upper limb ergometry, resistance training and use of functional electrical stimulation to augment cardiovascular response

- Participation in a regular, vigorous exercise or wheelchair sports program can improve health status, functional independence as well as decrease in physician visits per year, re-hospitalisations, and medical complications over time

References

- American Spinal Injury Association (ASIA) Learning Centre Materials – International Standards for Neurological Classification of SCI (ISNCSCI) Exam, 2015 Worksheet.

- Kirshblum SC, et al. International standards for neurological classification of spinal cord injury. J Spinal Cord Med 2011;34(6):535–546.

- Consortium for Spinal Cord Medicine. Prevention of Thromboembolism in Spinal Cord Injury, 2nd ed. Paralyzed Veterans of America, Washington, DC, 1999.

- McKim DA, et al. Home mechanical ventilation: a Canadian Thoracic Society clinical practice guideline. Can Respir J 2011;18(4):197–215.

- Consortium of Spinal Cord Medicine. Bladder management for adults with spinal cord injury: a clinical practice guideline for health-care providers. J Spinal Cord Med 2006;29(5): 527–573.

- Abrams P, et al. The standardisation of terminology of lower urinary tract function: report from the Standardisation Sub-committee of the International Continence Society. Neurourol Urodyn 2002;21(2):167–178.

- Bryce TN, et al. International Spinal Cord Injury Pain (ISCIP) Classification: Part 2. Initial validation using vignettes. Spinal Cord 2012;50(6):404–412.

- Paralyzed Veterans of America Consortium for Spinal Cord Medicine. Preservation of upper limb function following spinal cord injury: clinical practice guidelines for health care professionals. J Spinal Cord Med 2005; 28(5): 434–470.

- Braddom RL, et al. (Eds). Physical Medicine and Rehabilitation, 4th ed. Elsevier Saunders, Philadelphia, 2011.

- Frontera WR, et al. (Eds). DeLisa's Physical medicine and Rehabilitation: Principles and Practice, 5th ed. LWW, Philadelphia, 2010.

Appendix 1. Projected functional outcome for complete tetraplegics

Domain	C1-C4	C5	C6	C7	C8-T1
Feeding	Dependent	Independent with adaptive equipment after set up	Independent, may need adaptive equipment	Independent	Independent
Grooming	Dependent	Minimal assistance needed with equipment after set up	Some assistance needed to independent with adaptive equipment	Independent with adaptive equipment	Independent
Upper body dressing	Dependent	Assisted	Independent	Independent	Independent
Lower body dressing	Dependent	Dependent	Assisted	Some assistance needed to independent with adaptive equipment	Independent
Showering	Dependent	Dependent	Independent to some assistance needed with equipment	Some assistance needed to independent with equipment	Independent
Bed mobility	Dependent	Assisted	Assisted	Independent to some assistance needed	Independent
Weight shift Independent with power	Dependent in manual WC Assisted unless in power WC	Independent	Independent	Independent	
Transfers	Dependent	Maximum assistance	Some assistance to independent on level surface	Independent with or without board for level surfaces	Independent
Wheelchair propulsion	Dependent in manual wheelchair; independent with power wheelchair	Independent to some assist in manual WC, with adaptation on level surface; independent with power wheelchair	Independent with manual wheelchair with coated rims on level surface	Independent – except over curbs and uneven terrain	Independent

Appendix II. Potential outcome for complete paraplegics

	T2-T9	T10-L2	L3-S5
ADL	Independent	Independent	Independent
Bowel and bladder care	Independent	Independent	Independent
Transfers	Independent	Independent	Independent
Ambulation	Standing in frame, tilt table or standing WC Therapeutic ambulation	Homebound ambulant with orthoses Trial of limited community ambulation	Community ambulation possible
Orthoses	Bilateral KAFO forearm crutches or walker	KAFO with forearm crutches	KAFO or AFO with walking stick/ crutches

5
Traumatic Brain Injury Rehabilitation

ZENG Shanyong, YAP Giok Mei Samantha, CHUA Sui Geok Karen

Introduction

Traumatic brain injury (TBI) is a major cause of death and chronic disability worldwide and in the under-35 age group. There are 3 peaks in occurrence: in those aged < 5 years, 21–35 years and > 65 years. Males outnumber females by 4:1 in the younger subgroup and this ratio equalises in the elderly subgroup.

TBI is defined as an alteration in brain function, or other evidence of brain pathology, caused by an external force. Primary injuries from TBI include mass effect from subdural haematoma, diffuse axonal injuries and brain contusions commonly affecting the base of the frontal lobe and tips of temporal lobes.

Classification of TBI severity

Table 1. Classification of TBI severity.

	Mild	Moderate	Severe
Admission GCS	13–15	9–12	3–8
Coma duration	< 30 min	30 min–24 hours	> 24 hours
Post traumatic amnesia (PTA) duration	< 24 hours	1–7 days	> 7 days
Others	No focal neurologic deficits	Some deficits likely; patients often quite functional	Severe deficits likely

TBI rehabilitation assessment

Objectives: to classify injury nature, delineate motor, sensory, visual and other neurologic impairments, classify severity of injury, prognosticate short and long term outcomes and elucidate medical complications

Rehabilitation history

A detailed history should be taken from family, patient where possible and available medical records.

- Age at injury: rehabilitation outcomes are worse in older adults > 55 years of age

- Premorbid functional level and cognitive reserve (vascular risks, diabetes mellitus, education level, vocational capacity, need for appliances, level of community independence)

- Risk factors for TBI: past history of TBI, seizure disorder, uncontrolled psychiatric illness (e.g. schizophrenia), alcohol or substance abuse, prior diagnosis of dementia, frequent falls, learning disability

- Etiology of injury: motor vehicle accident, falls (level ground vs. fall from height), blunt or sharp assault, sports injury, blast related, etc.

- Mechanism of injury: closed injury (most TBI) vs. penetrating injury (e.g. gunshot wound, stab wounds) vs. blast injuries

- Any associated polytrauma: visceral injury, spine or pelvic, long bone fractures, spinal cord injury, soft tissue or ligamentous injury)

- Depth of coma: admission Glasgow Coma Scale score (GCS) (post resuscitation): lower admission GCS scores are associated with worse outcome. Concomitant central nervous system depressants such as alcohol, major tranquilisers, drug overdose can confound admission GCS

- Length of coma (defined as time from TBI till ability to open eyes and follow motor commands. Operationally this refers to GCS score > 8)

- Duration of post traumatic amnesia (PTA): duration from time of accident till ability to form continuous memory of ongoing events and includes duration of coma. Patients remain disorientated and amnesic for day to day events

- Duration of memory loss prior to injury (retrograde amnesia)

- Summary of medical course and treatment so far (cranial surgeries, peripheral injuries, length of ICU stay and acute stay, length of intubation and ventilation, tracheostomy, seizures, sepsis, bladder or bowel complications, cardiopulmonary complications and venous thromboembolic events, ventriculoperitoneal shunt)

- For polytrauma or surgical patients: summary of surgeries, weight bearing status, duration of collar/braces/splints, wound care

- Current medications, plans for other treatments (radiotherapy or chemotherapy post tumour excision, duration of antibiotics and elective cranioplasty)

Physical examination

- Objectives: detect TBI related neurological (motor, sensory, coordination, visual auditory, olfactory, gustatory) deficits, neurobehavioural deficits, trauma related physical losses and complications related to TBI (spasticity, movement disorder, cranial nerve deficits, loss or joint range of motion and prolonged immobility)

- To assess for cognitive impairment, both arousal and awareness level must be first determined

- Arousal can be assessed by any spontaneous eye movement, GCS and the absence/presence of sleep-wake cycle. Subsequently, finger pressure can be used to elicit pain for response

- Awareness can be elicited by any non-reflexic visual movement. Check for visual alerting response, visual fixation, visual tracking. Ability to follow one-step commands (grip finger, release finger, give thumbs up)

- Higher cortical function can be subsequently assessed

- Aphasia. Look for word-finding difficulties, semantic/phonemic paraphasia, jargon aphasia

- Unispatial neglect. Look for any gaze preference, check line bisection test

- Hemianopia. Assess visual field. In minimally conscious patients, can be assessed by visual threat to eye fields

- Attention, memory, concentration. Subjective assessment with mini-mental state examination and Montreal Cognitive Assessment (MOCA).

- Physical impairments can be directly due to neurological effects of TBI and effects of polytrauma or prolonged immobility

- It is advisable to adopt a systematic head to toe approach in diagnosis:
  - Surgical wounds. Check cranial surgical wounds for discharge, collections, wound dehiscence
  - Cranial nerve palsies. Most commonly affected nerves are CN I,

VII, VIII followed by CN II, III, IV, VI. Lower cranial nerves rarely affected. Check for relative afferent pupillary defect, doll's eye reflex, eye movement and hearing

- Swallowing. Bedside water swallow test and check for bolus awareness

- Speech. To look for dysphonia/dysarthria/aphasia/apraxia

- Neck. Assess for any concurrent cervical spine injury as spinal cord injury and traumatic brain injury can occur together (10–15%)

- Skeletal survey. Assess for any concurrent rib/spine/pelvis/hips/long bones fracture

- Neuromuscular examination. Assess for tone/spasticity. Look for any motor/sensory deficits. Assess coordination and balance. Gait examination is essential

- Problems related to prolonged immobility: postural hypotension, bladder distension (check post void residual urine volumes), rectal distension, decubitus ulceration, joint contractures (measure joint range of motion), deep vein thrombosis screen (clinical, D dimer assay, venous Doppler ultrasound)

- Nutritional status: weight, height, BMI, skin fold thickness, serum albumin, haemoglobin

Predictors of functional and neurobehavioural outcome

There are several poor clinical predictors of outcome:

- Depth of coma (GCS < 8) on admission

- Duration of coma > 24 hours, length of PTA > 14 days
  - PTA assessment tools include
    - GOAT: Galveston Orientation and Amnesia Test
    - WMPTAS: Westmead Post Traumatic Amnesia Scale
    - O-Log: Orientation Log

- Unequal pupil size

- > 55 years of age

Assessment of neurobehavioural impairments after TBI

- Ranchos Los Amigos Cognitive Functioning Scale (RLAS)
- The RLAS is a common neurobehavioural scale with description of functional, behavioural and cognitive levels to guide management team

Summary of RLAS scale

Level I: no response

Level II: generalized response

Level III: localized response

Level IV: confused, agitated response

Level V: confused, inappropriate, non-agitated response

Level VI: confused, appropriate response

Level VII: automatic, appropriate response

Level VIII: purposeful, appropriate response

Level IX: purposeful, appropriate, stand-by assistance on request

Level X: purposeful, appropriate, modified independent

Medical issues in traumatic brain injury

1. **Post traumatic seizures (PTS):** seizures occurring after TBI believed to be causally related to the TBI often occurring within the first week, provoked by TBI

2. **Post traumatic epilepsy (PTE):** recurrent unprovoked seizures occurring 24 hours apart which are a life-long complication of TBI

   - 80% of PTE starts within the first 2 years post TBI
     - Incidence correlates with TBI severity and amount of intracerebral blood
     - Incidence: 4% to 53%
     - Highest incidence after penetrating TBI, especially after gunshot wounds (53%)

- May present as focal or generalised seizures, status epilepticus or atypically with recurrent, episodic or severe cognitive, behavioural and affective changes
- Risk factors for PTE include
    - Age > 65 years
    - Chronic alcoholism
    - History of PTS
    - Penetrating TBI (gunshot wounds, bone fragments, foreign bodies)
    - Focal neurological deficits
    - Depressed skull fractures
    - Presence of cerebral contusions and lobar haemorrhages
    - Severe TBI
- Early seizure (within first week after TBI) increases risk of late seizures (> 1 week post TBI), hence prophylaxis is recommended
    - Prophylaxis with phenytoin reduces risk of early PTE from 14.2% to 3.6% but no benefit between day 8 and 2 years post TBI
    - Treatment with anti-epileptics should not routinely be used beyond the first 7 days after injury
- Commonly used agents for PTE include Carbamazepine, Valproate and Levetiracetam
- General recommendation for duration of treatment is 12–18 months

3. **Post-traumatic agitation after TBI**
    - Subtype of delirium occurring after TBI within the period of PTA
    - Characterised by excesses of behaviour, including one or more of the following: motor restlessness or akathisia (physical agitation, wandering, rocking, rubbing, scratching, thrashing), increased verbal output (screaming, shouting, vulgarities, hyperverbosity), emotional lability (crying, laughing, rapid changes of mood) and aggression towards self or others (hitting, boxing, throwing objects, sexually directed behaviours)
    - Classification and objective measurements of agitation can be made by

- RLAS level IV (prior to patient emerging to higher levels of RLAS V and VI)

- Agitated Behaviour Scale: a 14-item scale, rated on 4 levels, which objectively measures aspects of agitation such as lability, disinhibition, aggression and restlessness

- Management includes a search for reversible causes such as pain, metabolic derangements, sepsis, seizures, new intracranial lesions, medications

- Treatment includes behavioural, environmental modification and neuropharmacology (beta blockers, anti-convulsants, anti-depressants, anti-psychotics)

4. **Paroxysmal sympathetic hyperactivity (PSH)**

- An uncommon condition characterised by tachycardia, tachypnoea, hypertension, diaphoresis and hyperthermia due to excessive release of epinephrine and norepinephrine

- PSH episodes can occur several times per day and last for minutes or hours

- Mixed autonomic hyperactivity is another subset involving the parasympathetic nervous system with the following symptoms: bradycardia, bradypnoea, hypotension, hiccups, and excessive lacrimation

- PSH can occur spontaneously or with external triggers such as:
  - Pain
  - External stimulation, noxious stimuli
  - Body turning
  - Tracheostomy suctioning
  - Bladder or bowel distention

- PSH is a diagnosis of exclusion and secondary causes such as sepsis, pulmonary embolism, pain or dehydration must be excluded

- Proposed diagnostic criteria (observation confirmation 4 out of 6 symptoms):
  - Fever greater than 38.3°C
  - Tachycardia with 120 beats per minute or more

- ◆ Hypertension with systolic blood pressure more than 160 mmHg or pulse pressure higher than 80 mmHg
- ◆ Tachypnoea with respiratory rates higher than 30 per minute
- ◆ Excessive sweating
- ◆ Severe dystonia
  - ■ Treatment options include
    - ◆ Propranolol (PO 10–20 mg BD to Q6H)
    - ◆ Clonidine (PO 0.2–1.2 mg/day in divided doses)
    - ◆ Baclofen (PO 10–20mg TDS, max 70–80 mg/day)
    - ◆ Morphine (PO 10–30 mg Q4-6H; IV 2.5–10 mg Q4-6H)
    - ◆ Bromocriptine (PO 1.25 mg BD initially, titrated up to 10–40 mg/day)
    - ◆ Dantrolene (PO 25 mg BD-Q6H up to 400 mg max)
    - ◆ Lorazepam (IV/PO 2–4 mg Q6-8H)

5. **Endocrine issues**
   - ■ Post-traumatic hypopituitarism
   - ■ Cranial diabetes insipidus
   - ■ Hyponatremia
     - ◆ Cerebral salt wasting
     - ◆ Syndrome of inappropriate antidiuretic hormone secretion

6. **Spasticity**
   - ■ Please see chapter 14, Practical Approach to Spasticity

Functional outcome after TBI

Using the Glasgow Outcome Scale (GOS), 22% remained vegetative, 42% severely disabled, 25% moderately disabled and 10% achieved good recovery levels. Hence, 35% achieved substantial independence at home and partial independence in the community at 1 year.

Disorders of consciousness (DOC)

A proportion of survivors of acquired brain injury may experience prolonged disturbance in consciousness following emergence from coma. Classification of DOC include coma, vegetative state (VS) or minimally conscious state (MCS).

Table 2. Classification of disorders of consciousness.

	Coma	Vegetative state (VS)	Minimally conscious state (MCS)
Consciousness	No	No	Partial
Spontaneous eye opening	No	Yes	Yes
Sleep-wake cycle	No	Yes	Yes
Visual tracking	No	No	Yes/Inconsistent
Purposeful motor activity	No	No	Yes/Inconsistent
Yes/No responses, verbalisation, gestures (communication)	No	No	Inconsistent

Differential diagnoses of MCS

- Locked in syndrome

- Akinetic mutism

- Severe ascending motor paralysis with intact cognition (e.g. Guillain–Barre syndrome, botulism)

Standardised evaluation tools for DOC

- Coma depth (GCS) and duration

- Disability rating scale

- GOS

- Coma recovery scale-revised (CRS-R)

- Coma/near coma scale

- Others include evoked response potentials, quantitative EEG, functional MRI

Prognosis for DOC

Table 3. Prognosis for DOC.

	Recovery of consciousness
Unconscious > 1 month	33% by 3 months 46% by 6 months 52% by 1 year
Unconscious at 3 months	35% recovered consciousness at 1 year
Unconscious at 6 months	16% regained consciousness at 1 year

Rehabilitation of DOC

Rehabilitation strategies include:

1. Sensorimotor regulation

- Physical rehabilitation strategies should be started early and intensively, including:
    - Management of hypertonia, prevention of contractures, neuromuscular management (spasticity interventions, passive range of motion exercises, splinting, serial casting)
    - Communication aids using alternative augmentative communication (AAC) devices
- Structured sensory stimulation (SSS)
    - Titrate exposure to sensory stimuli to altered sensory threshold levels. Exposure is heightened or constrained in accord with baseline response levels (e. g. diminished auditory responsiveness may be exposed to high intensity auditory stimuli). In those with exaggerated auditory startle reflexes, exposure to ambient auditory stimuli (background music, beeping alarms) would be minimised

2. Neuromodulation

- Normalising neurophysiologic disturbances accompanying brain injury
- Include pharmacologic interventions, deep brain stimulation (DBS)

Cognitive rehabilitation in brain injury

Cognitive problems are common after a traumatic brain injury and cognitive rehabilitation aims to improve (or restore) cognitive functioning, allowing participation in activities which may be affected by difficulties in one or more cognitive domains.

Cognitive deficits include:

(a) Attention and concentration

- Attention underpins all aspects of cognition
- Mild impairments can restrict other processes such as capacity for new learning
- Impaired attention may be more pronounced early in recovery after TBI and improve months later

- Common complaints include mental slowing (reduced information processing speed), trouble following conversation, loss of train of thought, difficulty attending to two things at once, inability to concentrate for more than a few minutes and distractibility

(b) Learning and memory

- Most common symptom after TBI and most apparent during early intervals of retrograde amnesia and PTA
- Difficulties with learning and memory after emergence from PTA often persists

(c) Executive functioning

- Higher cognitive functions are primarily governed by the frontal lobe
- Frontal lobe functions include insight, awareness, judgment, planning, organisation, problem solving, multi-tasking and working memory
- Executive functioning enables a person to engage in independent and purposeful behaviours successfully

(d) Language and communication

- Communication problems stem from difficulties understanding and expressing information
- One may present with excessive talking, repeating oneself, rambling and having difficulty keeping to the point and inability to understand and appreciate sarcasm, jokes and irony

Cognitive rehabilitation interventions may be:

(a) Restorative — remediation of memory deficits

- Restore specific impairments that may underlie a range of everyday problems via retraining eg. drill and practice and computer based assisted training

(b) Compensatory — behavioural compensation or functional adaptation

- Overcome impairments that cannot be modified
- Use of external compensatory aids such as calendars (diaries, smartphones, tablets and mobile devices), lists and internal memory aids such as rehearsal, visual imagery and usage of mnemonics for memory and executive functioning

(c) Environmental (manipulation of environment or task)

- Maximise performance of daily tasks eg. quiet environment, reduce distracters, simplify tasks, chunking of large pieces of information, extra time for tests

(d) Behavioural

- Use of feedback and reinforcement for maladaptive behaviour (positive and negative reinforcements)
- Implementation of strategies such as verbal and written prompt by family members to monitor and use in the home and community

Medications for cognitive remediation in TBI

- Different medications are used to improve cognition in TBI
- These can be divided broadly into catecholaminergic stimulants, catecholaminergic non-stimulants and cholinesterase inhibitors
- Minimise or remove sedating or cognitively-impairing medications, regulate sleep-wake cycles before commencing neurostimulants
- Start low and go slow when starting medications for TBI remediation
- Catecholaminergic stimulants
  - Methylphenidate used predominantly for deficits of mental processing speed and attention span; given 5 to 30 mg/day in 2 divided doses; does not lower seizure threshold and hence can be used in patients with high risk of seizures
  - Monitor for sympathetic overstimulation effects
- Catecholaminergic non-stimulants
  - These include dopaminergic activities like amantadine, carbidopa/levodopa and bromocriptine. Amantadine has very good evidence for improving arousal and emergence from minimally conscious state. Monitor for postural hypotension and gastrointestinal side effects
- Cholinesterase inhibitors
  - These include donepezil, rivastigmine and may be used to improve memory in TBI. Monitor for seizures and gastrointestinal side effects

6
Geriatric Rehabilitation

PALANIAPPAN K

Introduction

- Fastest growing population of persons requiring rehabilitation services are adults over 65 years of age. This is because of the ageing population in Singapore and the rest of the world

- In Singapore, the proportion of adults aged 65 and older is projected to increase from 8.8 % (2009) to 18.7 % (2030) over the next 20 years

- There is a progressive increase in the prevalence of disability with age as there is higher incidence of common conditions (e.g. osteoarthritis, stroke and hip fractures) causing physical disability

- Geriatric rehabilitation is thus an important field with increasing demand in Singapore

- Major goal of rehabilitation programs for older people is to assist them to manage personal activities of daily living (ADL) without the assistance of another person. If this is not possible, the goal is to minimise the need for external assistance through the use of adaptive techniques and equipment. It is important for medical practitioners who work with older people to be able to recognise both a person's need for rehabilitation and his or her potential to benefit from it

Criteria for selection

- A major consideration is the ability to benefit from rehabilitation

- Prime determinant of this is the severity of the presenting disability and premorbid functional status

- Severe cognitive impairment is a risk factor for less favourable response

- Older people with minor disability related to health conditions such as knee osteoarthritis/wrist fractures can also benefit from rehabilitation, usually on an outpatient or domiciliary basis

- Chronological age per se should not be a factor in determining participation in rehabilitation

Assessment

- Assess premorbid function using standardised instrument, e.g. Barthel Index (besides the patient, speak to family and also patient's family physician)

- Severity of present level of disability

- Medical comorbidities identified and managed. For example, cardiac failure, anaemia, urosepsis can negatively impact patient's ability to participate and benefit. Reduce delirium episodes and ensure optimal pain management for effective participation in rehabilitation. Ensure patients are as medically stable as possible, but stability is not a pre-requisite

- Cognitive impairment: standardised assessment tool, e.g. Mini Mental State Examination which is a screening tool, not a diagnostic tool. Interpret results carefully as language issues can affect cognitive assessment. The patient should be able to follow one-step commands and has sufficient recall of instructions to participate in rehabilitation. Even if the patient has severe cognitive impairment, rehabilitation should still be considered. The goals of rehabilitation can be environmental and behavioural modification, maintenance physical therapy, and caregiver training

- Vision and hearing assessed and corrected to maximise older person's ability to participate

- Motivation and therapy tolerance. Assess mood using standardised assessment questionnaire, for example Geriatric Depression Scale (GDS). Determine whether treatment or further psychiatric assessment is required. Although rehabilitation in itself helps with depression, patient must be willing to participate

Management
The rehabilitation process

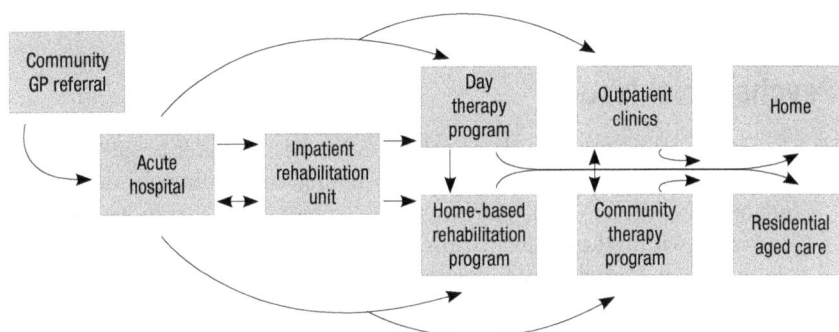

Fig. 1. Process and settings of rehabilitation from referral to discharge (adapted from Cameron and Kurrle, 2002).

- Have specific goals—primary aim of rehabilitation is most commonly mobility and self-care without the assistance of another person

- Coordinated multidisciplinary team of nurse, physical therapist, occupational therapist, medical social worker, psychologist and physician. Regular team meetings involving patient and family in goal setting

- No time specified care pathways because comorbidities can complicate and interrupt rehabilitation

- Monitor achievement of specific goals progress (e.g. Functional Independence Measure, Barthel Index)

Exercise and physical activity for older adults

- Exercise is key to the prevention and treatment of chronic diseases and disability

- Physical inactivity is a significant risk factor for development of many chronic conditions that impacts functional mobility in older adults (e.g. heart disease, depression, type 2 diabetes, osteoporosis, etc.), and it also increases the risk of additional disability in individuals with pre-existing chronic conditions e.g. chronic back pain, balance problems and falls, stroke, arthritis, and Parkinson's disease

- Slippery slope of ageing (fun → function → frailty → failure) — ageing is not an automatic descent into frailty. A continuous amount of high-level physical activity is the key to maintaining a quality of life that allows individuals "to die young at a very old age"

- Types of exercises for older adults—strength and balance training, aerobic (measurement of target heart rate, cardiac index, rate of perceived exertion etc. Refer to chapter 8, Cardiopulmonary Rehabilitation), aquatic, stretching, plyometrics, and Tai Chi

Psychosocial issues

- Recognise and resolve psychosocial issues by assisting older people to adapt to consequences of a disabling illness. Listening, counselling and quiet encouragement are important. Note that complex intergenerational conflict may arise within the family because of caregiver fatigue and burden, so discussion and provision of appropriate support services may help

- Communication: fostered by formal meetings with family and family physician (face to face or by telephone) to update and finalise rehabilitation goals

Rehabilitation of older people in community settings

- Contemporary rehabilitation practice is not confined to traditional inpatient rehabilitation units; it also occurs in the community and other non-hospital settings, and involves general practitioners/physician (e.g. geriatrician or rehabilitation physician supervising multidisciplinary care)

- Rehabilitation for older people should be provided on an episodic rather than on a continuing basis. Once goals have been achieved or it is clear that only limited progress is achievable then patient should be discharged from rehabilitation. Often older people will have multiple episodes of episodic rehabilitation due to their chronic disabling medical condition

Healthcare directives, alternate decision maker and ethics

- A multi-faceted approach to aged care is adopted by Singapore, which has a ministerial committee on ageing. It also has laws to support caregiving by families in the form of family or childcare leave. It passed the Maintenance of Parents Act in 1996 to allow impecunious old parents to sue their children for maintenance. Singapore has enacted 2 laws on advanced medical directives and surrogate decision-making

- The Singapore Advance Medical Directive (1996) allows persons to state in advance that they do not wish to have extraordinary medical treatment should they be terminally ill, on the point of death, and unable to communicate. The practical application has been limited because doctors seldom ask whether patients have signed an advanced medical directive, and the level of take up by the public has been low

- The Singapore Mental Capacity Act (revised edition 2010) allows individuals to appoint a surrogate decision maker for healthcare decisions should they lose their capacity to make those decisions in the future. However, the surrogate does not have the power to make decisions on life-sustaining treatment or treatment to prevent a serious deterioration in the patient's health. The doctor makes those decisions in the patient's best interests

- Also there are various laws to protect the older persons from elderly abuse, e.g. The Women's Charter protects the elderly (whether male or female) against family violence. In situations where the elderly is of unsound mind, any person related by blood or marriage can apply to the court for managing the elderly and his affairs through The Mental Disorder and Treatment Act

- Familiarity with these laws is helpful for healthcare staff managing the older persons and advising them on various options should they require them

- Ethical concerns and sources of conflict abound in regard to the rehabilitation of geriatric patient such as in discharge planning, use of restraints, end of life care and long-term care. Although a detailed review of these issues is beyond the scope of this chapter, it is imperative that healthcare staff who work with elders should be sensitive to these issues, understand the ethical principles and incorporate moral values into the decision-making process

- In addition to the traditional bioethics principles and codes of ethics, clinicians should be mindful of reflective practice, incorporate care and compassion, and avoid ageism when making decisions that impact on the lives of older persons, their families and society

Specialised rehabilitation programmes for older people

Amputee rehabilitation

- Older people have higher incidence of lower limb amputations than other age groups because of the effects of vascular disease. The principles of lower extremity amputee rehabilitation in older people are similar to other disabling illnesses

- Aim for distal amputation preserving knee joint as much as possible, control stump edema with bandaging, prevent contractures, start strengthening exercises early after surgery and use of temporary prosthesis during mobility training (e.g. pneumatic post amputation mobility aid, fit definitive prosthesis and discharge when semi-independent using prosthesis or wheelchair)

Mental health and ageing

Depression

- Assessment scales: Geriatric Depression Scale, Center for Epidemiological Studies, Depression, Patient Health Questionnaire-9, etc

- Unique features of depression in the older adult include unexplained or aggravated aches and pains, hopelessness, helplessness, anxieties and worries, memory problems, weight loss, loss of feeling of pleasure, slowed movement, irritability, lack of interest in self-care, tiredness and listlessness

- One factor consistently associated with depression in older people is physical illness (e.g. stroke is consistently associated with depression)

- Factors contributing to increased risk of depression in physical illness can be biological (such as endocrine abnormalities, effects of medication, physical consequences of systemic and/or intracerebral disease) or psychological (e.g. sense of loss associated with serious medical illness, effects on body image, self-esteem, sense of identity and impaired capacity to work and maintain relationships)

- Management
    - Pharmacotherapy
    - Psychotherapy (Cognitive Behavioural Therapy, problem solving, interpersonal and psychodynamic therapies)
    - Exercises. Either resistance or aerobic type is beneficial in reducing depression

Cognitive decline

- Decline in some aspects of intelligence in later years of life should not affect function in the non-cognitively impaired individual. The degree of neuroanatomical changes that occur and subsequently affect cognition variably represents the continuum of normal cognition to disease

- Preservation of cognition in old age includes engaging in cognitively stimulating activities, physical activities and having a rich social network. In a 9-year follow up of a healthy ageing sample in Sweden by Karp et al. (2006), individuals who were active in any of the key dimensions of health, i.e. cognitive, physical or social, had lowered dementia risk. Those who were active in 2 or all 3 dimensions had the lowest risk of all. However, longer term follow-up studies are needed to assess whether or not participation in cognitive training programs and/or adoption of cognitively stimulating lifestyles forestalls the expression of clinical dementia or impacts neurobiology in disease-modifying ways

- Given the limitations in current knowledge, it can be difficult to answer patients' questions about the "best" things to do to increase the odds of healthy cognitive ageing. However, the risks of harm from recommending a cognitively active lifestyle, or enrolment in a memory training class, are small

Mild cognitive impairment

- Factors affecting rate of progression of mild cognitive impairment to dementia include severity of cognitive deficits, APOE ε4 carrier status, atrophy on MRI, functional imaging modality (FDG PET scans showing pattern of Alzheimer's disease), CSF markers compatible with Alzheimer's disease and positive molecular imaging of amyloid. Presently, no pharmacological treatment is approved for treatment of mild cognitive impairment

Delirium

- Common risk factors include age older than 65 years, severe illness, dementia, poor vision, urinary catheters, polypharmacy and low albumin. Management includes treatment of reversible causes e.g. pain, avoidance of physical restraints, early mobilisation, adaptive equipment for vision and hearing, and encouraging contact with familiar surroundings and people

Dementia

- Common causes include Alzheimer's, Lewy body disease, vascular and frontotemporal dementia. Less common causes are traumatic brain injury, alcohol, normal pressure hydrocephalus, anoxia and infection

Assessment

- Mental status assessment of attention, immediate and delayed recall, remote memory, executive function, depression and cognitive screening (e.g. Mini Mental State Examination, Mini-Cog Assessment and neuroimaging to rule out unexpected pathology)

Management

- Goal: to improve quality of life and maximise function by enhancing cognition and addressing mood and behaviour.

- Identify and treat comorbid physical illnesses (e.g. hypertension, diabetes mellitus)

- Promote brain health by exercise, balanced diet, stress reduction

- Avoid anticholinergic medications

- Limit as required psychotropic medication use

- Specify and quantify target behaviours

- Assess and monitor psychiatric status

- Intervene to decrease hazards of wandering

- Monitor physical environment for safety (e.g. stairs)

- Advise patient and family with regards to driving

- Establish and maintain relationship with patient and family

- Advise patient and family about sources of care and support, financial and legal issues, and advance directives, including establishing surrogate decision maker

- Consider referral to hospice (Reisberg Functional Assessment Staging (FAST) Scale = 7

(Adapted from American Geriatrics Society: Dementia Diagnosis 2010)

- Pharmacology: cholinesterase inhibitors, vitamin E (caution in those with cardiovascular disease because > 400 IU is associated with increased mortality). In the presence of severe behavioural and psychological symptoms associated with dementia (BPSD), neuropeptide modifying agent, antipsychotics, anxiolytics, and mood stabilisers can be considered

- Behaviour: Antecedent-Behavioural-Consequences (ABC) strategies and environmental management (consistent, safe and secure environment). Effective strategies to improve function and modify behaviour, according to the American Academy of Neurologists guidelines (2010), include (a) reducing urinary incontinence by scheduled toileting, behaviour modification, prompted voiding, (b) increase functional independence by graded assistance, practice and positive reinforcement and (c) reduce problematic behaviour by playing music, particularly during meals and bathing and walking or other forms of light exercise

- Exercise: physical activity is associated with better cognitive function and less cognitive decline in later life (Lautenschlager et al., 2009). The Seattle

Protocols: evidence based programme of task specific and less cognitive-demanding exercises designed for older adults with dementia

- Key to reducing caregiver stress management: education regarding strategies to deal with behavioral problems, including role playing, enhancing ADL abilities, reinforcement with practice, home visits, phone calls and encouraging self-care with pleasurable activities and health promoting behavior

- Depression and dementia: trial regimen of antidepressants may provide information for a clearer diagnosis. PHQ-9 may be useful for differentiation

Falls

- Consequences: pain, functional decline, loss of confidence, institutionalisation

- Comprehensive fall risk assessment: ask the following fall risk screening questions:
  - Does the patient present with a fall?
  - Has the patient had > 2 falls in the last 12 months?
  - Does the patient report having trouble with walking/gait and/or balance?

(Adapted from the summary of the updated American Geriatrics Society/British Geriatrics Society clinical practice guidelines for prevention of falls in older persons by American Geriatrics Society (2011))

- If answer is positive to any of the above screening questions, obtain relevant history, physical examination, cognitive and functional assessment. Determine risk of falls through noting prior history of falls, medications, gait (timed up and go test and gait speed), balance and mobility (Berg Balance scale, Romberg's test, single leg stance, and functional reach), visual acuity (plus contrast sensitivity, depth perception, and visual field restriction), any other neurological impairments such as somatosensory impairment (vestibular, proprioception, vibration, and cutaneous sensation), sensory integration testing (computerised dynamic posturography), neuromuscular testing (range of motion, endurance, and muscle strength), heart rate and rhythm, postural hypotension, feet and foot care and environmental hazards. Initiate multicomponent intervention to address identified risks and prevent falls by minimizing medications, providing individually tailored exercise programmes, treating visual impairments including cataracts, managing postural hypotension, managing heart rate and rhythm abnormalities, supplementing with vitamin D, managing footcare problems, modifying the home environment and providing education and information

- However, if the answer is negative to all the above screening questions but there is a single fall reported in the past 12 months, evaluate patient's gait and balance. If there are abnormalities in gait or unsteadiness is identified, assess the patient and initiate multicomponent interventions as above. Always reassess patient periodically

Management

- Main goal: maximize independence in mobility and function and prevent further falls.

  - Environmental modification—such as changes in lighting, handrails, floor surfaces, beds, bathroom and use of assistive devices (hip protectors, footwear with sensory cues for impaired sensation)

  - Medical strategies—review medications to reduce sedation and postural hypotension, address visual problems with specific types of glasses and ophthalmology consultation for cataracts. For example, vitamin D supplements have been found to decrease rate of falls but not fall risk in nursing homes, weight-bearing or standing exercises with medications for osteoporosis, and incontinence management

  - Rehabilitation strategies—the American Geriatrics Society and the British Geriatrics Society recommends multicomponent exercises including strength, balance coordination e.g. Tai Chi, and gait training. Physiological manoeuvres such as active movements of lower extremities prior to moving from sit to stand and use of elastic pressure stockings or an abdominal binder are beneficial in decreasing orthostatic events

Frailty

- Definition: widely accepted Cardiovascular Health Study definition as follows:

- 3 or more of the following characteristics: unintentional weight loss of 10lbs or more in a year, self-reported general feeling of exhaustion, weakness, slow walking speed, low levels of physical activity

- Causes are multifactorial and include sarcopenia (loss of muscle strength, power and functional quality), dependency, low oxygen from atherosclerosis, cognitive impairment, undernutrition, decreased balance and fear of falling

- To assess severity: Modified Physical Performance Test
- Treatment: resistive exercises, balance and endurance training

Osteoporosis and minimal trauma fracture, e.g. vertebral compression fractures

- Goal: to achieve movement and function in a pain free and competent manner within optimal postural alignment
- Evaluation: the presence of a previous minimal trauma fracture is the most important risk factor; bone density measurement (DEXA scan), pain measurement, total body alignment, range of motion, strength of core muscles, respiratory function, static and dynamic balance assessment
- Management: besides pharmacological treatment for pain and osteoporosis, therapeutic exercises to correct faulty posture (strengthening, endurance and stretching exercises for trunk and extremities), respiratory exercise, ADL retraining, manual therapy to increase flexibility and decrease pain, external supports (taping, brace, 4-wheeled walker, orthotics) to assist better posture, thermal agents and electrotherapeutics. Bone stimulating exercises like "osteoporosis dance", a weight-bearing exercise programme that focuses on standing balance, coordination and muscle endurance and walking while maintaining optimal posture
- Outcome assessment—pain score, flexible curve measurements, prone trunk lift with arms by the side, Oswestry Disability Index, kyphotic index

Osteoarthritis (OA)

- Refer to Chapter 11, Adult Joint Reconstruction Rehabilitation

Continence management

- Bladder and bowel incontinence among older persons is common and often treatable. Unfortunately, embarrassment and inadequate knowledge of treatment or treatment options prevent many older persons from reporting incontinence to doctors. Older persons who live at home may eliminate or reduce trips outside the home due to care needs and embarrassment. Moreover, older persons with urinary incontinence are at increased risk of falls due to wet floor, drug effects (confusion and postural hypotension), urgency (patient hurries to void), disturbed sleep pattern due to nocturia. Perineal skin complications may include severe infections and even sepsis in the frail elderly

- Faecal incontinence: causes include faecal impaction, loss of normal continence mechanism (e.g. local neuronal damage causing loss of sensation or muscle tone, anorectal trauma/sphincter disruption, impaired neurological control, e.g spinal cord injury, previous injury from damage occurring during childbirth, stroke), problems that overwhelm normal continence mechanism (e.g. diet, infection, drugs), psychological and behavioural problems (e.g. severe depression, dementia, stroke)

  - Management: obtain careful history from patient and medical record. Physical examination includes abdominal palpation for colon distension, per rectal examination, neurological examination, assessment of mobility, hygiene and mental functioning. Diagnostic tests may include stool cultures, barium enema, manometry and defecography. Treatment depends on underlying cause and severity of incontinence. Diet management (e.g. increasing fluid and fibre intake), bowel management and training may involve medications and a toileting schedule. Neuromuscular re-education, including biofeedback, and pelvic musculature strengthening

- Urinary incontinence: basic workup is aimed at identifying possible reversible causes (DIAPPERS mnemonic: Delirium, Infections, Atrophic urethritis and vaginitis, Pharmaceuticals, Psychologic disorders, Excessive urine output, Restricted mobility, Stool impaction). If no reversible cause is identified, then the incontinence is considered chronic. The next step is to determine the type of incontinence (urge, stress, overflow, mixed, or functional) and the urgency with which it should be treated, an assessment of other medical problems that may contribute to incontinence (e.g. bowel, back, gynaecologic surgery), a discussion of the effect of symptoms on the patient's quality of life, a review of the patient's completed voiding diary, a physical examination (for neurological disease, abdominal mass, pelvic organ prolapse, prostate examination), and, if stress incontinence is suspected, a cough stress test. Other components of the evaluation may include laboratory tests, pad testing, measurement of postvoid residual urine volume and urodynamic studies. If the type of urinary incontinence is still not clear, or if red flags such as hematuria, obstructive symptoms, or recurrent urinary tract infections are present, referral to a urologist or urogynecologist should be considered

  - Management: guided by underlying cause and severity of incontinence. Some causes are reversible and easily treats transient incontinence. If functional incontinence, environmental manipulation, absorptive products, external collection devices, behaviour therapy, use of bladder relaxants and indwelling catheter in selected patients can be considered. Pelvic floor muscle (Kegel) retraining (including biofeedback, strengthening exercises, endurance exercises), medications to prevent unwanted detrusor contractions or to increase muscle tone, bladder training to gradually increase time interval between voids till an acceptable voiding schedule is reached (including patient education, diet counseling, scheduled voiding, positive reinforcement, urge suppression techniques), transvaginal electrical stimulation and, surgical urinary diversion can be considered. There is growing evidence to support recommendations for lifestyle measures such as weight loss, caffeine reduction and fluid management for urge incontinence. For sphincter related causes, options include Kegel exercises, oestrogen treatment, alpha agonists, bulking agents to increase bladder outlet pressure by reducing urethral lumen, surgical procedures e.g. slings/artificial sphincter. For overflow incontinence, consider surgical correction, clean intermittent catheterisation, indwelling catheters in patients who cannot self-catheterise, and who are not good candidates for surgical correction. General measures include perineal skin care and frequent change of absorptive products like diapers and pads

Recommended reading

- Cameron ID, Kurrle, SE. Rehabilitation and older people. Med J Aust. 2002;177(7):387–391.

- Guccione A, et al. Geriatric Physical Therapy, 3rd ed. Elsevier, Missouri, 2012.

- Kauffman T, et al. A Comprehensive Guide to Geriatric Rehabilitation, 3rd ed. Churchill Livingstone, New York, 2014.

- American Academy of Neurologists. Detection, Diagnosis and Management of Dementia Guidelines. Accessed 28 June 2016. Available at: http://tools. aan.com/professionals/practice/pdfs/dementia_guideline.pdf.

- American Geriatrics Society. A Guide to Dementia Diagnosis and Treatment. Accessed 28 June 2016. Available at: http://unmfm.pbworks. com/f/American+Geriatric+Society+Dementia+Diagnosis+03-09-11.pdf.

- Summary of the updated American Geriatrics Society/British Geriatrics Society clinical practice guideline for prevention of falls in older persons.

Accessed 28 June 2016. Available at: http://www.americangeriatrics.org/files/documents/health_care_pros/JAGS.Falls.Guidelines.pdf.

- Karp A, Paillard-Borg S, Wang HX, et al. Mental, physical and social components in leisure activities equally contribute to decrease dementia risk. Dement Geriatr Cogn Disord 21(2): 65–73, 2006.

- Lautenschlager NT, Cox KL, Flicker L, Foster JK, van Bockxmeer FM, Xiao J, Greenop KR, Almeida OP. Effect of physical activity on cognitive function in older adults at risk for Alzheimer disease: a randomized trial. JAMA. 2008 Sep 3;300(9):1027–1037.

7

Lower Limb Amputee Rehabilitation: Basic Grounding

VICTOR Somu, TJAN Soon Yin

Introduction

Singapore has one of the highest lower extremity amputations in the world. Approximately 4 amputation procedures are done per day at the various public hospitals in Singapore as shown by data available in public media. Vascular causes of lower limb amputation (diabetes, peripheral vascular disease) are more common than trauma or tumors.

Amputee rehabilitation is best studied by remembering the **phases of rehabilitation** and also the **roles of the multidisciplinary team.** Table 1 shows the key phases, milestones, tasks and time line using the example of vascular below knee amputation (the most common type of major limb amputation).

Table 1. Milestones and important tasks for vascular below knee amputee rehabilitation.

	Pre-prosthetic		
	Pre-operative	Immediate post-operative	Pre-casting
Milestones	Patient activation	Superficial wound healing	Stump ready for casting
Main tasks	-Education, prognostication and goal setting -Start reconditioning -Control comorbidities	-Wound management and on time suture removal -Pain management	Stump shaping
Ideal time line for completion (all dates from day of amputation)	Days before amputation	3 weeks	6 weeks

Prosthetic			
	Prosthetic gait training	Community re-integration	Maintenance
Milestones	-Proficient care of prosthesis -Safe walking in controlled environment	Resume community activities	Self care ability and know when to engage rehab team
Main tasks	Gait training and prosthetic adjustment for final lock-tight, foam-up	Community rehabilitation including return to work and/or driving assessment and rehabilitation	-Save up for next prosthesis -Join amputee support groups -Proficient care for underlying medical conditions
Ideal time line (all dates from day of amputation)	3 months	6 months or earlier	3 years

There are significant overlaps of the tasks from one phase to another. An example is the need for adequate pain management and continued reconditioning throughout all the phases and also the need to continue educating and motivating the patient and significant others. The **goals of amputee rehabilitation** are not just returning to independent living (Activity domain of the International Classification of Function) and active community participation (Participation domain of the International Classification of Function), but also **on-time progression through the phases** which can only be achieved via **good coordination of the multidisciplinary team.** Fig. 1 shows the usual members of the amputee rehabilitation team.

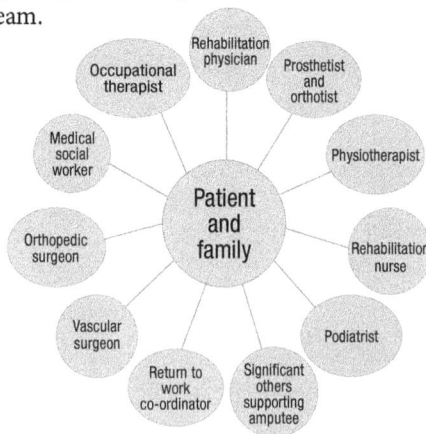

Fig. 1. Members of typical amputee rehabilitation team.

The **common roles of a rehabilitation physician** are as follow:

- Holistic assessment of amputee's medical and functional status

- Prevention and on time follow up of complications

- Understand needs of amputee in order to prescribe appropriate prosthetic system and follow up

- Set rehabilitation goals and initiate rehabilitation

- Support other rehabilitation team members

- Educate and explain prognostication to patient and significant others

- Advocate for suitable integration back to society

- Medical legal representation on insurance and compensation cases

Prognosticating functional recovery and goal setting in amputee rehabilitation

A patient who has had an amputation loses more than a limb. Using the ICF (International Classification of Function)–WHO framework, we can understand the amputee's decreased ability to transfer and ambulate (disability) and because of these disabilities, the amputee may become home bound and lose his or her vocational and leisure roles in the community (handicap). With this framework in mind, the most important prognosticating factors for an amputee (using the example of a lower limb amputee) will be his or her premorbid mobility level, his or her current mobility level and also his or her desire or need for future participation.

Expressed in a formula, it will look like:

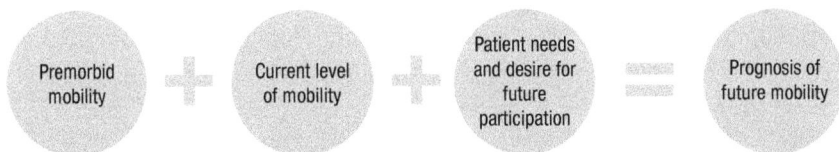

Premorbid mobility + Current level of mobility + Patient needs and desire for future participation = Prognosis of future mobility

The most commonly used categorisation for amputee mobility is the Medicaid/Medicare amputee mobility category (also known as amputee K classification) shown in Table 2.

Table 2. Medicaid/medicare amputee ambulation category.

K level	Definition	Expressed as
K0	Unable to use prosthesis to stand, transfer and move from point to point	Non ambulatory
K1	Able to ambulate short distances on level ground in a home or controlled environment	Home bound ambulator
K2	Able to ambulate with fixed cadence on level ground in the community slowly and with caution	Limited community ambulator
K3	Able to ambulate with variable cadence over uneven terrain and traverse slope and stairs. A typical community ambulator.	Unlimited community ambulator
K4	Able to use prosthesis to perform heavy manual task and or participate in sports requiring running	Heavy manual user or sports user

Another commonly used lower limb amputee mobility assessment tool is the Amputee Mobility Predictor Index (AMPI). AMPI provides a more objective and detailed testing of a lower limb amputee's ability to ambulate.

Coming back to the formula above, an amputee who was K2 prior to the amputation but had an acute myocardial infarction or developed other complications immediately post operation resulting in longer than expected bed bound period, may have his future goal and prognosis lowered to K1 and a carer may be needed upon discharge from inpatient rehabilitation. Conversely, an amputee who did not develop significant post-operative complication and receive proper and on time rehabilitation will be highly likely to return to his or her premorbid K status even though he or she has lost a limb.

It should be noted that the equation above offers a platform for assessment of the amputee at an early stage post amputation. Mobility post amputation is a composite function determined by level of amputation (proximal amputation carry worst prognosis), status of remaining leg (whether it can adequately weight bear), cardiovascular status (due to increased energy expenditure ambulating with non-natural leg), cognitive ability (learning a new gait pattern with safety in mind), upper limb function (due to the need to use a walking aid at least in the beginning of prosthetic gait training) and also presence or absence of stump pain.

It is worthwhile to note that for an amputee aiming to return to work, K3 is the usual mobility target for walking training with a prosthesis. A K3 amputee will be able to traverse uneven grounds and walk with variable cadence—giving him or her the ability to use public transport and travel to work. Having said this, there are amputees who have successfully re-integrated into the workplace using a suitable wheelchair and appropriate support from employers.

Pre-operation phase

Amputations are seldom carried out as an emergency operation immediately after admission. It is necessary, first and foremost, to stabilise the patient's medical status, and also to explain the need for amputation and to obtain consent from the patient. The patient should be referred to the rehabilitation team or suitable explanation given on post-operative prognosis and rehabilitation care plan. A thorough explanation will not only facilitate consent taking, but alleviate fear and uncertainty for the patient and family promoting early active participation in subsequent amputee rehabilitation. The key tasks in the post-operative phase are found in Table 3.

Table 3. Key tasks during pre-operation phase.

Tasks
Explaining prognosis, exploring rehabilitation goals and plans
Assessment of functional status especially presence of deconditioning
Teach bed exercises, teach use of mobility aid (e.g. walking frame)
Pain management (enrolling the help of acute pain management team if necessary)
Explore and refer to medical social worker for social and financial help

Immediate post-operation phase

The main tasks in this phase are wound management and pain control (see Table 4). Both are supremely important as done poorly, it will delay the amputee's progress into the subsequent phase of rehabilitation and more importantly, may hamper the extent of functional recovery. For example, poor pain control during the peri-operative phase has been implicated in sustained pain post amputation and poor wound management can result in need for repeat operation and prolonged hospital stay. The use of Removable Rigid Dressing (RRD) also showed evidence of controlling post-operative stump edema and shorten duration for wound healing. However, the care of a RRD and its usage should be taught to all involved in post-operative wound care, including the ward nurses, amputees and their caregivers.

Table 4. Key tasks during immediate post operation phase.

Tasks
Pain relief (stump pain, phantom pain, pain of other body areas—usually MSK origin). Teach pain desensitisation techniques
Wound management (emphasis on use of wound product and dressing change regime via protocol and in coordinated fashion)
Use of Removable Rigid Dressing (RRD) to control stump edema and prevent delay on wound healing, elevate stump while lying down
Contracture prevention (e.g. for below knee amputee, prevent prolonged knee flexion while using wheel chair)
Balance training, sit to stand training, ambulate out of bed supervised by physiotherapist

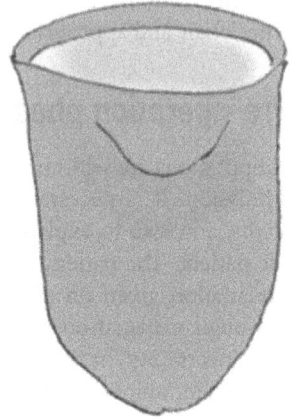

Fig. 2. Removable Rigid Dressing (RRD).

Pre-casting phase

Key tasks in this phase are all centered on getting the stump ready for early casting of prosthetic socket (see Table 5). A stump suitable for casting should be correctly shaped (not bulbous), without edema (checked by applying manual pressure via examiner's finger), not overtly sensitive to pain, have skin that is not dry, wound should be well healed and no underlying adhesion present. Although the focus is on stump condition, the amputee should be ready for gait training as the immediate task following making of the prosthesis is none other than walking training. By this phase, the patient should already be ambulating short distances with walking frame using the remaining leg and reconditioned to tolerate the rigor of starting prosthetic gait training.

Table 5. Key tasks during pre-casting phase.

Tasks
Stump shaping using compressive stump shrinker (wound healed and no ischemic contraindication), e.g. Juzo
Stump massage for desensitisation
May start weight bearing and short distance walking with preparatory prosthesis or pneumatic training prosthesis
Cardiovascular reconditioning to continue
Exercise for musculoskeletal system especially for promoting truncal control
Explore need for financial assistance and to refer to medical social worker if needed

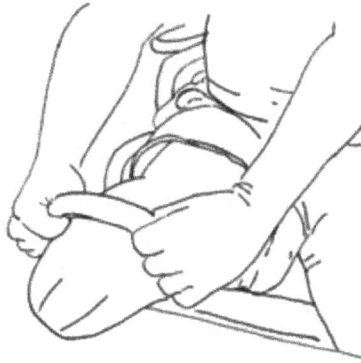

Fig. 3. Correct donning of stump compression stockings is necessary to ensure edema control and good shape of the stump.

Assessment of first visit amputee at amputee clinic

A common question asked by healthcare colleagues is "when to refer patient to the amputee clinic". The answer in short form, is when the patient is ready for casting of the prosthesis (i.e. when the patient has successfully passed through the above 3 phases). In a vascular below knee amputee that has progressed in ideal fashion, this can be as early as 6 to 8 weeks post amputation. A full-fledged amputee clinic, however, will be able to advise the patient and primary team on the ideal timeline (earlier or later) due to wound problems, persisting pain or marked deconditioning and provide consultation to determine the best plan for rehabilitation. Patients requiring higher level prosthesis or specialised prosthesis may be seen earlier too in order to explore funding for more expensive variants of artificial limb. The five important questions to ask during a first visit consult are listed in Table 6, together with check list of what to ascertain when seeing the patient.

Table 6. Important check list during first visit at amputee clinic.

1. Is the patient a functional walker?	Premorbid K classification, cardiovascular status, ability to stand and walk with aid
2. Is patient ready for prosthetic casting?	Wound healed, absence of stump edema and pain. Remaining leg able to safely tolerate walking.
3. What type of prosthesis system should be made?	K classification of walking goal, cost consideration, special need for vocational and leisure use

| 4. What is the complete rehabilitation plan? | Need for close monitoring, logistic constraints (e.g. transport), any financial constraint needing medical social worker help, any need for referring to occupational therapists for driving rehabilitation |
| 5. Is there any system integration issue that needs to be considered? | Diabetes mellitus control, need for earlier vascular surgery consult for remaining limb ischaemia, need for stump refashioning. System coordination if wait time is unacceptably long |

Prosthetic gait training phase

The focus of this phase is to train the amputee to walk with his prosthesis (see Table 7). This is also a good stage to reinforce the importance of looking after the remaining leg, and also start to explore what kind of community participation the patient desires (e.g. return to work). This phase can last between one to three months, depending on factors including the logistics of arranging outpatient appointments with therapists and also the gap between patient's current condition and planned K level/ambulatory goals.

Table 7. Key tasks during prosthetic gait training phase.

Tasks
Gait training with prosthesis
Training on care and use of prosthesis
Continued reconditioning
Reinforce care of remaining leg

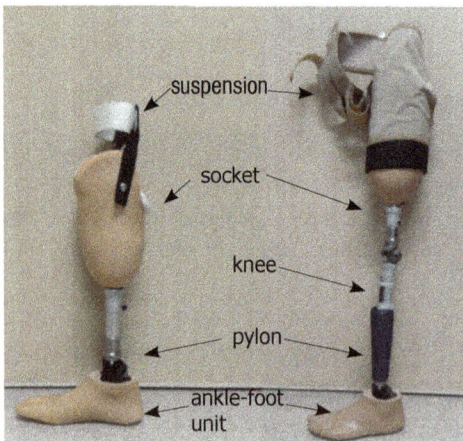

Fig. 4. Parts of a below knee amputation and above knee amputation prosthesis.

Trouble shooting prosthetic use problem

Trouble shooting starts with identifying the cause and it may involve more than one member of the multidisciplinary team and occasionally may take more than one session. More often than not, the issue at hand may be a combination of any of the following categories listed in Table 8 which shows a simplified approach to trouble shooting.

Table 8. Examples of common prosthetic usage problems and their causes.

	Common examples
Equipment (prosthesis) problem	Length discrepancy, socket fit (too loose or too tight) issues, over riding brim, too much or too little flexion at joint, failure to relieve pressure or sensitive areas on stump
User problem	Stump volume changes (fluid overload), shrinkage of stump, skin problem, uncontrolled stump pain
Usage problem	Wrong technique of wearing the prosthesis, inadequate weight shift to prosthetic side, failed attempt to repair prosthesis by user, poor care of non-waterproof components

Using the example of a below knee (trans-tibial) stump, Fig. 5 illustrates the pressure sensitive and pressure tolerant areas around the stump.

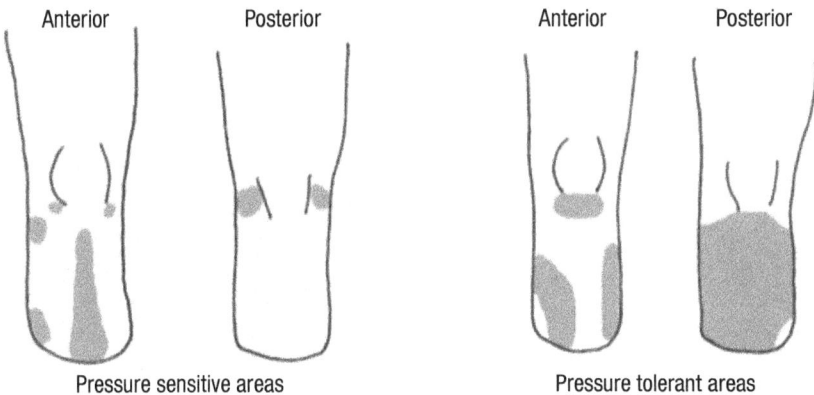

Anterior   Posterior   Anterior   Posterior

Pressure sensitive areas   Pressure tolerant areas

Fig. 5. Pressure sensitive areas: fibula head, directly over amputation scar, hamstring insertions. Pressure tolerant areas: patella tendon, calf, both sides of the shin.

Community reintegration phase

By now the amputee should be proficient in self-care at home. Treatment emphasis now shifts to enhancing participation in the community. A community/ home rehabilitation team is invaluable in this aspect. Medical social worker and occupational therapists also play prominent roles here. The doctor representative in the team may need to advocate for the amputee with the help of the employer (if the amputee was holding a job). Medical reports and insurance claims should be completed by this phase.

Table 9. Key tasks in the community reintegration phase.

Tasks
Prosthetic usage problem solving
Community rehabilitation to maximize integration into society
Vocational rehabilitation, driving rehabilitation

Maintenance phase

The usual warranty for common prosthetic components is three years. Some components may require more frequent changes (e.g. silicone liners). The cost of life time maintenance should be educated early so that the amputee or significant others do not misunderstand that a prosthetic system can last a life time. The presence of a prosthetic support group consisting of existing prosthetic users and their caregivers can also be very useful for motivating the new amputee.

Table 10. Key tasks in the maintenance phase.

Tasks
Link new amputee with support group
Educate and support amputee on need and cost of subsequent prosthetic renewal
Provide appropriate upgrade and troubleshooting for enhanced participation in sports and vocational pursuits
Lifestyle changes including smoking cessation, dietary modification and cardiovascular risk factor control

Conclusion

Amputee rehabilitation encompasses all the processes aiming not just at treating the impairment (giving amputee a prosthesis), but improving activity performance and ultimately participation and return of quality of life. The patient will progress through phases of rehabilitation, helped by a well-coordinated multidisciplinary team. The key to success lies in each team member knowing what is needed in order to best help the amputee at each phase—the axiom "do the right thing at the right time" is most appropriate in amputee rehabilitation.

8

Cardiopulmonary Rehabilitation

VADASSERY Shaji Jose

Introduction

Endurance training is beneficial for those with physiologic, functional and/or psycho-social deficits related to diseases of the cardiovascular and pulmonary system. This improves the patient's ability to generate adenosine triphosphate (ATP) aerobically and thus improve aerobic fitness.

Indications

Aerobic capability training can be considered in those diagnosed with ischemic heart disease, myocardial infarction, stable angina, congestive heart failure, post-cardiac and valvular surgeries.

Pulmonary rehabilitation benefits patients who have symptoms or functional limitations from chronic respiratory diseases, despite best medical management. These include fatigue, respiratory and associated cardiac impairments, reduced exercise tolerance as well as psychological issues such as anxiety, depression, etc.

Goals and benefits of cardio-pulmonary rehabilitation

- Establish a patient-controlled and safe aerobic exercise program
- Reduction in dyspnea, anxiety and depression
- Maximises cardiovascular and pulmonary capacity and mechanical efficiency
- Provide guidelines for safe activities and work by energy conservation strategies
- Improve quality of life and activities of daily living (ADLs), mobility and social activities
- Control risk factors for coronary artery disease (CAD)
- Decreased frequency of hospitalisations

Contraindications for cardiopulmonary exercise programs

- Unstable angina, active pericarditis, myocarditis or recent embolism
- Severe aortic stenosis, severe pulmonary hypertension, recent myocardial infarction
- Uncontrolled diabetes, symptomatic congestive heart failure
- Acute systemic illness or fever
- Resting systolic blood pressure (BP) > 200 mmHg and diastolic BP > 100 mmHg
- Orthostatic BP drop or drop of > 20 mmHg during exercise training
- Sinus tachycardia (> 120 bpm)
- Uncontrolled atrial or ventricular dysrhythmia, 3rd degree atrioventricular (AV) block
- Resting ST displacement (> 3 mm)
- Neurologic and orthopedic problems that may interfere with training

Assessment for cardiorespiratory fitness

A detailed examination to assess

- Risk factors, symptoms or signs of active cardiac or pulmonary disease
- Premorbid and current activities and endurance levels
- Cognitive and behavioural status, mood, vision, nutritional status
- Physical impairments that may affect exercise training
- Laboratory data, electrocardiogram (ECG) or echocardiographic abnormalities to institute special precautions as needed
- Optimisation of pharmacologic management

Determine baseline exercise capacity

- A 6 (or 12) minute walk test evaluates exercise tolerance. It measures the distance an individual is able to walk over a total of six minutes on a hard, flat surface.
- VO2 max: the gold standard for assessment of aerobic capability; it is the maximal oxygen consumption during incremental exercise. This is typically

done, by a specialist, on a motorised treadmill and is a measure of the maximum intensity of exercise that can be sustained.

- In special populations with stroke or spinal injuries, alternative tests like cycle or arm ergometry are alternatives.

For those with underlying respiratory disease:

- Spirometry
- Baseline Dyspnoea Index (BDI) or Transition Dyspnoea Index (TDI)

There is a linear relationship between heart rate (HR) and percentage of VO2 max. An exercise of at least moderate intensity (i.e. 40% to 60% of VO2 max) can be considered at the start of rehabilitation programme with incremental increases. A lower target can be planned for higher risk groups.

Steps of cardiopulmonary rehabilitation

Rehabilitation integrates into the medical continuum of care and should be tailored to the needs of each individual.

Cardiac rehabilitation

It is divided into three sequential phases:

Phase I: inpatient training phase

- Understand patient's previous activities and life roles, as well as current goals
- Establish modifiable risk factor reduction strategies
- Establish level of the risk for development of complications
- Early ambulation and ADL training under supervision and monitoring
- Alleviation of anxiety and reassurance
- Patient education regarding rationale for treatment and exercises
- Prescription of exercises for activity and work after discharge

Phase II: outpatient training phase

- Continue the goals of phase I
- Establish the strategies and a safe level of exercise tolerance
- Cardiovascular conditioning and fitness via an aerobic exercise training program that is monitored

- Control of modifiable risk factors using psychosocial, pharmacologic and lifestyle interventions

- Achieve an early return to work

Educate the patient to self-monitor for the appropriate level of exercise, work, or activities via heart rate (HR) monitoring and/or rating of perceived exertion (e.g. Borg scale) and psycho-social support to reduce anxiety and depression.

Phase III: maintenance phase in a community-based setting

- Continue the goals of phase II

- Patient self-monitored continuation of the aerobic exercise program to avoid overexertion

- Risk-reduction strategies and activity/work modifications

- Periodic evaluation to monitor the patient's progress and tolerance

These should result in improvements in VO2 max, lowering of HR for a given workload, reduced systolic BP and have beneficial peripheral effects on improvement of O2 utilisation by skeletal muscle. It will also result in reduction of anxiety and depression and improved coping mechanisms.

Pulmonary rehabilitation

(a) Respiratory muscle training: Inspiratory muscle training: generally initiated at low intensities then gradually increased to achieve 60 to 70% of maximal negative inspiratory pressure (PImax). Breathing training strategies: pursed-lip and diaphragmatic breathing.

- Pursed-lip breathing: involves a nasal inspiration followed by expiratory blowing against partially closed lips, avoiding forceful exhalation. This strategy is often unconsciously used by patients with COPD to enhance exercise tolerance during periods of dyspnea and increased ventilatory demand. Pursed-lip breathing does reduce respiratory rate, minute ventilation, and carbon dioxide level, and increases tidal volume, arterial oxygen pressure, and oxygen saturation

- Diaphragmatic breathing: consciously expand the abdominal wall during inspiratory descent of diaphragm

(b) Endurance training: start based on baseline exercise capacity with incremental level of training.

Types:

- Sustained exercise: 20 to 30 min two to five times a week, at levels of 60% of the maximal work load or

- Interval training: 2 to 3 min of high-intensity (60 to 80% maximal exercise capacity) training alternating with equal periods of rest

- Dynamic exercises are preferred over isometric exercises as cardiac output is higher with lesser increment in systolic BP and reduction in diastolic BP due to peripheral vaso-dilatation in the former

(c) Methods of endurance training:

- Upper extremity endurance training: supported arm exercises with ergometry or unsupported arm exercises by lifting free weights and stretching elastic bands

- Lower extremity endurance training: stationary cycle exercise, treadmill walking, or ground-based walking

Many activities of daily living require more arm work than leg work. Therefore, persons with coronary artery disease are advised to use their arms as well as their legs in exercise training. The arms respond like the legs to exercise training both quantitatively and qualitatively, although ventilatory oxygen uptake is less with arm ergometry. Although peak heart rates are similar with arm and leg exercise, heart rate and blood pressure response during arm exercise is higher than leg exercise at any submaximal work rate. Therefore, target heart rates are designated 10 beats per minute lower for arm training than for leg training.

(d) Education forms an integral part of any successful cardiopulmonary rehabilitation programme. This includes: energy conservation and work simplification techniques—assist patients in maintaining ADLs, home management, shopping, and job performance. Methods include paced breathing, which is based on principles of reducing breath-holding and timing the respiratory cycle with physical activities, optimising body mechanics, advanced planning, prioritisation of activities, and the use of assistive devices

- Airway clearance

- Coping and anxiety management

- Smoking cessation

- Nutrition

(e) Follow up assessment: Improvement of functional status and symptoms should be assessed at regular intervals using any of the following:

- Chronic respiratory disease questionnaire—self or interviewer administered

- 6 or 12 min walking tests (minimal clinically meaningful increase in the 6-minute walk test distance is about 54 m)

- Borg scale of perceived exertion: a rating of exertional and overall dyspnea

Exercise prescription

Model 1:

(a) Frequency: 2 days per week for 6–8 weeks;

(b) Intensity: low to moderate (low: 11–12 on Borg Scale; 50–65% maximal HR (HRmax) in test; 10–25 beats increase in resting HR; moderate: 13–14 on Borg Scale; 60–75% of HRmax in test; 20–35 beats increase in resting HR, duration: 30 min of activity daily at a similar level of Borg or HR.

Model 2:

70–85% of HR on exercise test, 20–40 min, 3 days per week for 12 or more weeks.

How to calculate the target HR:

(a) Maximal heart rate (HRmax) method:

HRmax = 220 – age (standard deviation of +/- 10 beats/min)

70% to 85% of HRmax approximates to 55% to 75% of VO2max

(b) Heart rate reserve (HRR) method (Karvonen method):

HRR = HRmax – HRrest

Low target HR = 50% HRR + HRrest

High target HR = 80% HRR + HRrest

Rating of Perceived Exertion (Borg scale): It is a subjective grading of how hard individuals feel during exercise. Uses a 6–20 grade score where 11 denotes "fairly light", 13 denotes "somewhat hard" (approximates to 60% of VO2 max) and 15 denotes "very hard" (approximates 80% of VO2 max). Use of rating of perceived exertion is considered an adjunct to monitoring HR in those

- where HR response to exercise may have been altered because of medications or

- individuals who have difficulty with HR method

Monitoring:

- Watch the percentage change of the maximum heart rate (maintain < 120 bpm)

- Watch for any bradycardia or inadequate heart rate increase in response to exercise

- Dyspnea ratings: Borg scale, Baseline Dyspnea Index (BDI) or Transition Dyspnoea index (TDI)

- Consider the need for supplemental oxygen to maintain SPO2 > 90% (if PO2 < 55–60 mmHg)

- Discontinue exercise if chest pain, severe dyspnea or > 6 ventricular premature beats/min occur during exercise

Recommended reading

- Agency for Health Care Policy and Research. Cardiac Rehabilitation Guidelines Panel: Cardiac Rehabilitation. Clinic Practice Guidelines no. 17. Rockville, MD, AHCPR, 1995, AHCPR publication no. 96-0672.

- American College of Sports Medicine guidelines. 2005.

- Ornish D, Brown S, Scherwitz L, et al. Can lifestyle changes reverse coronary heart disease? The Lifestyle Heart Trial. Lancet 1990;336:129–133.

- Casaburi R, Petty TL (eds). Principles and Practice of Pulmonary Rehabilitation. W.B. Saunders, Philadelphia. 1993.

- Bausewein C, et al. Measurement of dyspnoea in the clinical rather than the research setting. Curr Opin Support Palliat Care 2008;2:95–99.

- American Thoracic Society Pulmonary Rehabilitation guidelines. 1999.

- Astrand P-O, Elblom B, Messin R, et al. Intra-arterial groups. J Appl Physiol 1965;20(2):253–256.

- Fletcher GF, Balady G, Blair SN, Blumenthal J.A statement for health professionals by the committee on exercise and cardiac rehabilitation of the council on clinical cardiology, American Heart Association 1996; 94: 857–862.

- Goble A, Worcester M. Best Practice Guidelines for Cardiac Rehabilitation and Secondary Prevention. Department of Human Service Victoria, Victoria, Australia. 1999.

9
Rehabilitation of Low Back Pain

YAP Eng Ching

Introduction and epidemiology

- Annual incidence of low back pain 5% to 10%

- 80% of population have back pain at some point in their lifetime

- It is the most common musculoskeletal condition and the second most common complaint after upper respiratory tract infection seen in general practice

Clinical anatomy

- Lumbar spine consists of 5 vertebrae with a lordosis angle of 30 to 50 degrees between lumbar 1 and 5 vertebrae

- Lumbar spine articulates inferiorly with the sacrum, which articulates with coccyx and a pair of innominate bones to form the pelvis

- A line across the top of both iliac crest passes between lumbar 4 and 5 vertebrae

- Posterior superior iliac spine (PSIS) is at the level of sacral 2 vertebrae

- Motion segment of lower back is a 3 joint complex: a large anterior inter-vertebral joint and 2 small posterior facet/zygapophyseal joints between the articular processes

Clinical biomechanics

- Lumbar disc pressure changes with body posture. If the disc pressure is 100% when standing:

  - Disc pressure decreases to 25% in recumbent posture

  - Increases to almost 150% when sitting

  - Almost 150% when standing and bending forward

- The above explains aggravation and relief of herniated disc symptoms in these postures.

Clinical biomechanics: lumbar flexion

- During lumbar flexion, cross sectional area of the spinal canal increases. Anterior elements of the lumbar spine: disc and vertebral body are loaded and stressed.

- Flexion compression injury of intervertebral disc or vertebral body, post menopausal osteoporotic vertebral fracture in the elderly may occur

- Flexion combined with rotation may result in various lumbar spine injuries

Clinical biomechanics: lumbar extension

- During lumbar extension, cross sectional area of spinal canal decreases.

- Posterior elements of lumbar spine, facet joint and pars body are loaded and stressed

- The lumbar spine is more stable in extension than flexion

Lower back muscle imbalance

- Imbalance of lower back muscles is often seen in lower back pain

- Global postural muscles such as erector spinae, quadratus lumborum and hamstrings are often hypertonic and overactive

- Local dynamic muscles such as multifidus, pelvic floor muscles, gluteus maximus and medius, are often hypotonic and lax

- Imbalance of lumbo-pelvic muscles predisposes the lower back to dysfunction and degeneration

Kinetic chain and degenerative cascade

- The musculoskeletal system is a dynamic and inter-related kinetic chain

- Dysfunction and injury of lower back may have ripple effect on proximal and distal segments in the kinetic chain, and lead to further injury and a cascade of degeneration

Pathophysiology of intervertebral disc

- Disc degeneration: loss of disc hydration and disc resorption within the annulus fibrosus

- Internal disc disruption: nuclear pulposus migrates into radial fissure in annular fibrosus, may initiate release of enzyme phopholipase A2 and activate inflammatory mediators

- Disc herniation: annular fibrosus is completely breached with gross herniation of nuclear pulposus; most commonly occurs at 30 to 40 years of age, majority at L5S1 level followed by L45 level; most of the symptoms usually resolve with conservative treatment in 6 to 12 months

Pathophysiology: lumbar degeneration

Degeneration of the lumbar spine results in the loss of disc hydration and narrowing of disc space, joint hypertrophy and osteophytosis. Lumbar stenosis most commonly occurs at L3L4 level.

Causes of low back pain

Low back pain is often due to vertebral dysfunction: Facet joints, intervertebral disc joint, the associated ligamentous and muscular attachments. Vertebral dysfunction is also known as mechanical back pain.

Other causes of back pain include: disc herniation and nerve root compression; degeneration of disc and facet and lumbar stenosis; traumatic and osteoporotic fracture; spondylolysis and spondylolisthesis; severe spine deformities and instabilities.

In many cases, the relationship of back pain to underlying structure and function remains controversial.

History

- Distribution pattern of back pain can be broadly divided into axial pain and radicular pain

- It is important to elicit the acute or gradual nature of pain onset; associated aggravating and relieving factors, and whether the pain is improving or worsening over time, with or without treatment

- Discogenic pain is often worsened by sitting; bending and lifting, and during Valsalva manoeuvre

- In central stenosis and pseudo-claudication, back and leg pain is aggravated by walking and relieved by forward flexion, sitting or squatting. It is also more painful walking downhill than uphill

- Though uncommon, non-spinal condition such as systemic, visceral, vascular, neurological disease may present with pseudo-spine pain

Red flags for sinister pathology

- Exclude cauda equina syndrome in back pain patients with saddle or bilateral lower limb signs or symptoms; bladder, bowel or sexual dysfunction

- Urinary retention is the most common complaint in cauda equina syndrome and it is a surgical emergency

- Exclude infection or tumor in the presence of systemic symptoms such as fever or weight loss; nocturnal and constant pain unrelated to body position; and pain unresponsive to treatment

Yellow flags: psychosocial factors for long term disability

- Affect: low negative mood; anxiety; depression; impaired sleep

- Belief and behavior: catastrophic thinking; fear and avoidance; sickness behavior; passive coping strategy; belief that pain and activity are uncontrollable and harmful; belief that pain has to be eliminated before returning to normal activities

- Work: unsupportive work environment; poor job satisfaction; pending claims or compensations

- Social: social withdrawal; lack of support; overprotective family; history of physical abuse, or substance abuse

Physical examination

- Look, move and feel

- In the screening examination, both quality and quantity of motion are important. They provide clinical information to the areas that require further evaluation

- Examine the global and postural muscles, e.g. erector spinae, quadratus lumborum, piriformis for myofascial trigger points

- Examine and exclude neurological deficits distal to the lumbar spine and in the lower limbs

Tests for sacroiliac joint (SIJ) dysfunction

- Gillet test: patient stands, raises one leg to 90 degrees and ipsilateral PSIS should rotate inferiorly. Restriction of this motion is considered abnormal

- Seated flexion test: patient sits and bends forward. Asymmetric cephalad motion of PSIS indicates SIJ dysfunction.

- FABER test: flexion, ABduction and External Rotation of the hip produces pain in dysfunctional SIJ on the contralateral side

- Gaenslen test: patient supine and contralateral hip flexion, dropping involved leg off bedside produces SIJ pain

- Iliac compression test: patient lying on side, downward force on iliac crest produces SIJ pain

- Yeoman's test: patient prone, hip extension and ilium rotation produces SIJ pain

Nerve tension tests

- Lasegue straight leg raise: sciatic pain when hip in flexion < 70 degrees; and pain is relieved by knee flexion and aggravated by foot dorsiflexion.

- Bowstring: when straight leg raise elicits sciatica, flex knee to reduce symptom and then apply pressure on popliteal fossa to reproduce symptom

- Crossed straight leg raise: sciatic pain down the contralateral lower limb is a sign of severe nerve root impingement

- Femoral stretch/reverse Lasegue straight leg raise: patient is prone and examiner passively extends hip with knee flexed to 90 degrees. Pain in anterior lateral thigh is a sign of femoral nerve root tension

- Slump test: radiating sciatic pain when seated with neck flexion, thoracic slump, knee extension and ankle dorsiflexion. The symptom is relieved by reversing the maneuver

Waddell signs of non-organic back pain

- Sensitive and tender back pain on light superficial palpation

- Non-anatomic sensory/motor abnormalities; widespread pain

- Simulation tests: low back pain on cranial axial loading; back pain on shoulder–pelvic rotation

- Distraction tests: seated and supine straight leg raise

- Over-reaction to testing and examination

Investigation and clinical correlation

- In the absence of red flags, further investigation is not indicated in the initial management of most cases of low back pain

- Imaging studies show static anatomy of the lumbar spine. Electro-diagnostic studies reveal dynamic physiology of muscle and nerve function

- Abnormal MRI scans are found in 25% of asymptomatic population and the prevalence of abnormal imaging rises with increasing age

- Abnormal finding on imaging scan may not be the source of pain. The clinician must correlate the history, physical examination, findings from other tests and treatment to determine the likely pain generator

- Imaging guided injection procedure may provide both diagnostic and therapeutic benefit to enhance the progress of rehabilitation

Management

- Majority of back pain can be managed conservatively

- Explain pain and help the patient understand why the back hurts can help improve daily function

- Absolute rest leads to de-conditioning. Relative rest is more appropriate

- Signs and symptoms of neurological dysfunction are not always due to anatomical nerve root compression. It can be due to physiological nerve root inflammation. Neurological complaint can also result from non-neurological dysfunction

- The goal of rehabilitation is not to cure pain. It helps to reduce pain intensity and frequency, improve daily function and enable self-management

Physical modalities

- Physical modalities such as heat, electrical therapy and traction may help as supplementary treatment of back pain. They are passive therapeutic modalities and their effects are usually temporary.

- Braces and corsets may help as a short term adjunctive treatment for back pain. However, prolonged use will lead to back de-conditioning

Back exercises

- Extension biased back exercises are often prescribed if back pain is from the anterior elements of the lumbar spine—inter-vertebral disc or vertebral body

- Flexion biased back exercises are often prescribed if back pain is from the posterior elements of the lumbar spine—facet joint or pars body

- Gluteal, core and active conditioning exercises help to rebalance back muscles and yield long term benefits

Medications

- Analgesics help to control back pain, reduce inflammation and dampen sensitization

- Commonly used analgesics for back pain include paracetamol, non-steroidal anti-inflammatory drugs and synthetic opiate analog such as tramadol.

- Adjuvant analgesics: anticonvulsants such as gabapentin and pregabalin dampen down central sensitization; antidepressants such as tricyclics (e.g. amitriptyline, nortriptyline) and serotonin–norepinephrine reuptake inhibitor (e.g. duloxetine) enhance central descending inhibition of neuropathic back pain

- The somnolent effect of analgesics and adjuvant analgesics help improve sleep and relieve muscle fatigue

Interdisciplinary approach

- Chronic back pain with de-conditioning, psychosocial issues and multiple barriers to recovery will benefit from a comprehensive interdisciplinary rehabilitation approach, active conditioning exercise program coupled with cognitive behavioral therapy to enable self-management and optimize function

Prognosis

- Back dysfunction often continues to persist even when the pain has resolved

- 90% of back pain subsides within 3 months but 80% of cases continue to have recurrent pain in the subsequent 1 to 2 years

- About 50% of back pain patients who missed work for 6 months return to work. Almost 0% of back pain patients who missed work for 2 years returned to work eventually

- 10% of back pain patients continue to suffer chronic residual symptoms

Recommended reading

- Stout A. Low back pain. Physical Medicine and Rehabilitation Clinics of North America 2010;21(4).

- Liebenson C. Rehabilitation of the Spine: A Practitioner's Manual, 2nd ed. Lippincott Williams & Wilkins, 2007.

- Haig A, Colwell M. Back Pain: A Guide for the Primary Care Physician. American College of Physicians, 2005.

10

Rehabilitation Approach to Common Cancer-related Problems

TAN Ping Ping

Cancer and its treatment can cause multiple impairments, activity limitations and participation restrictions. Common functional impairments include loss of motor control, cranial nerve deficits, cognitive and speech problems, swallowing problems and sensory loss. Due to the progressive nature of malignancies, rehabilitation goals may be divided into:

Restorative: to return to premorbid functions with minimal functional deficits

Supportive: to reduce functional difficulties and compensate for permanent deficits

Palliative: to eliminate or reduce complications

Preventive: understanding possible complications and early symptoms/ signs, pre-operative education and optimizing of function

Below are some of the common issues seen in cancer rehabilitation:

Cancer-related fatigue

- Cancer patients may experience loss of energy and impairment of physical functions.

- Fatigue may be a severe and activity limiting symptoms and is **not improved** by rest.

- Cancer fatigue is the most common symptom among advanced cancers but is common throughout the disease continuum.

Table 1. Fatigue in cancer: causes and management.

Causes and associations of cancer-related fatigue	Suggested treatment
Poor sleep quality	Sleep hygiene, medication
Medications (e.g. analgesic, anti-epileptics, beta-blockers, sedatives/ hypnotics, anti-depressants)	Medication/dosage reassessment
Pain	Assessment of pain generators, medication, therapy
Hormonal deficiency	Replacement if no contraindications
Distress (anxiety, depression, stress)	Support, counseling, medications
Anemia	Transfusion, investigation/ treatment into blood loss
Hypercalcemia	Correction
Inactivity, debility	Exercise
Malnutrition, dehydration	Supplements, appetite stimulants

Work up for cancer-related fatigue

- Need to exclude secondary causes of fatigue e.g. symptomatic anemia.

- As inappropriate rest, or inactivity may induce/worsen muscular catabolism, prolonged rest may aggravate the symptoms and lead to negative effects on self care and social activities.

- Factors contributing to impaired physical performance:
  - Decreased endurance
  - Decreased strength
  - Reduced nutritional status
  - Sleep disturbances
  - Biochemical changes secondary to disease and treatment

- Reduced psychosocial and emotional state
- Reduced level of physical activity

- Rather than prolonged rest, cancer patients should exercise appropriately. Other interventions include stress and nutritional management, energy conservation, activity/exercise program, diversional activity and appropriate rest/sleep patterns. The aim is to return to normal daily activities as soon as possible.

Goals of exercise prescription

- Regain and improve physical function, aerobic capacity, strength and flexibility
- Improve quality of life
- Improve body composition and image
- Improve cardiorespiratory, endocrine, neurological, muscular, cognitive and psychological outcomes
- Potentially reduce or delay recurrence of secondary primary cancer
- Reduce, attenuate and prevent long term and late effects of cancer treatments

General contraindications

- Extreme anemia or ataxia
- General injury risks/contraindications for/during exercise may include
    - Osteoporosis from bone metastasis and bone- wasting drugs
    - Peripheral neuropathy
    - Altered immune function
- Follow American College of Sports Medicine Guidelines for exercise prescription regarding cardiovascular and pulmonary contraindications to exercise
- Potential for adverse cardiopulmonary events may be higher in cancer survivors than age-matched comparisons (due to toxicity of treatment/late effects of malignancy)

Metastatic bone involvement

- Most consistent symptom: pain, most severe at night or upon weight bearing

- May cause neurological involvement, functional impairment and pathological fractures

- Skeletal metastases are rarely solitary

- Most common sites of involvement: axial skeleton, proximal femur and humerus

- Spinal involvement- most common in the thoracic spine, mostly extradural, mostly involving vertebral body anterior to spinal canal

Evaluation of bony metastasis

- May include:
  - Bone scan
  - X-rays
  - MRI when appropriate

- Treatment may include:
  - Operative management plus rehabilitation to restore mobility and self care
  - Radiotherapy

- During radiotherapy, bones are at increased risk of fractures (as a result of hyperemic softening of bone and necrosis of tumour cells, and complete ossification may not occur till 6 months or more)

- Would need weight bearing precautions and reduced load-bearing. May need assistive devices, orthosis and adaptive/compensatory strategies for mobility and self care

Criteria for prophylactic fixation

- Presence of significant functional pain

- > 50% destruction of cortical bone

- Useful staging systems include Harington's criteria and Mirel's criteria

- Is preferable over fixation of actual pathological fractures — shorter operative time, decreased morbidity, quicker recovery

Harington's criteria

- >50% destruction of diaphyseal cortices

- 50–75% destruction of metaphysis (>2.5cm)

- Permeative destruction of the subtrochanteric femoral region

- Persistent pain following irradiation

Mirel's criteria

Table 2. Mirel's criteria for prophylactic fixation.

Score → Variable ↓	1	2	3
Site	Upper limb	Lower limb	Peri-trochanteric
Pain	Mild	Moderate	Functional
Lesion	Blastic	Mixed	Lytic
Size*	< 1/3	1/3–2/3	> 2/3

*As seen on plain radiographs, maximum destruction of cortex in any view
Maximum possible score = 12
A score of 8 = a fracture risk of 15%
If a lesion scores 9 ≥ then prophylactic fixation is recommended prior to radiotherapy.

Malignant spine disease

- Common symptoms of spinal cord compression are pain, weakness, autonomic dysfunction, and sensory loss (including ataxia)

- May have bone pain secondary to bony destruction or pathological fractures

- Local pain may be due to stretching of periosteum, and may respond to radiation therapy

- Axial pain occurs with vertebral compression and/or collapse, and is secondary to mechanical instability. In many cases, surgical decompression with stabilisation and radiotherapy may be warranted. This would stabilise the diseased bone and allow for ambulation with pain relief

- Neuropathic pain may be due to root irritation and/or meningeal irritation sec to tumour infiltration

- The Spine Oncology Study Group defines spine instability as "loss of spinal integrity as a result of neoplastic process that is associated with movement-related (functional) pain, symptomatic or progressive deformity and/or neural compromise under physiological loads."

- There is no widely accepted definition of what constitutes an unstable spine. Older approaches were often based on clinical features, e.g. pain on movement that was not present during rest with supportive radiological features

- The stability of the thoracolumbar spine can be described using the 3 column model:

    - Spine is considered "stable" when only 1 column is involved except for the middle column

    - Spine is considered "unstable" when ≥ 2 columns are involved or middle column is severely affected

    - Spine is also "unstable" if > 20° angulation is present

- Higher predictors of spinal instability would include:

    - Subluxation/translation

    - Progression of deformity

    - > 50% vertebral body collapse

    - Bilateral facet joint destruction

    - Movement-related pain (functional pain) as opposed to rest pain

    - Areas of greater concern: occipitocervical, cervicothoracic, thoracolumbar junction

Consensus opinion (Spinal Instability Neoplastic Score)

Table 3. Spinal instability neoplastic score.

Component scores for clinical and radiologic findings	Score
Spine location	
Junctional (occiput: C2, C7-T2, T11-L1, L5-S1)	3
Mobile spine (C3-C6, L2-L4)	2
Semi rigid (T3-T10)	1
Rigid (S2-S5)	0
Pain relief with recumbence and/or pain with movement/loading of spine	
Yes	3
No (occasional pain but not mechanical)	1
Pain-free lesion	0
Bone lesion quality	
Lytic	2
Mixed lytic/blastic	1
Blastic	0
Radiologic spine alignment	
Subluxation/translation	4
De novo (kyphosis/scoliosis)	2
Normal alignment	0
Vertebral body collapse	
> 50% collapse	3
< 50% collapse	2
No collapse with > 50% body involvement	1
None of the above	0
Posterolateral involvement of spinal elements (facet, pedicle, costovertebral joint fracture replacement by tumour)	
Bilateral	3
Unilateral	1
None	0

A patient with a score of 7 or greater is considered at risk of spinal instability and surgical consult is warranted.

Functional prognostic predictors

- Pretreatment ambulatory status

- Slower development of motor deficits prior to treatment

- Radiosensitive tumours

Cancer and treatment related neuropathies

- Polyneuropathy may occur as a result of direct invasion, or part of a paraneoplastic process, or with chemotherapy

- Paraneoplastic neuropathy may be related to an autoimmune process, and may be sensorimotor in nature

- Chemotherapy associated peripheral neuropathy are generally distal, symmetric and length- dependent in a "glove- and stocking" distribution. Predominantly sensory symptoms with sensory axonal damage and reduced amplitude of the sensory nerve action potentials (SNAPs) in nerve conduction studies. Often dose-dependent. Symptoms may include numbness, paraesthesia and neuropathic pain

Table 4. Common chemotherapy drug implicated in peripheral neuropathy.

Class of drugs	Examples
Platinum based drugs	Cisplatin, carboplatin, oxaliplatin
Taxanes	Paclitaxel, docetaxel, cabazitaxel
Epothilones	Ixbaepilones
Plant alkaloids	Vinblastine, vinorelbine and etoposide
	Thalidomide, lenalidomide, pomalidomide
	Bortezomib, Carfilzomib

Common chemotherapy drugs implicated are shown in Table 4.

- Treatment measures may include:

  - Tricyclics (e.g. nortriptyline), antidepressants (e.g. duloxetine), and antiepileptics (e.g. gabapentin)

  - Adaptive strategies: energy conservation, orthotics, assistive/adaptive devices

  - Preventive strategies especially when lower extremities are involved (e.g. non-constrictive footwear, daily inspection of feet)

Lymphedema

- Lymphedema is swelling that occurs when protein rich lymph fluid accumulates in the interstitial tissues

Diagnosis

- The most common way to diagnose upper limb lymphedema is by taking circumferential measurements at specific bony landmarks. Differences of 2 cm or more may be clinically significant

Severity classification

- Stage I: pitting edema, increased upper limb girth, and increased heaviness. Spontaneously reversible

- Stage II: spongy consistency without pitting edema. Tissue fibrosis can then cause limb to harden and increase in size

- Stage III: lymphostatic elephantiasis, uncommon post breast cancer therapy

Common terminology criteria for adverse event (CTCAE)

- Grade 1: 5–10% interlimb discrepancy in volume or circumference at point of most visible difference; swelling or obscuration of anatomic architecture on close inspection; pitting edema

- Grade 2: more than 10–30% interlimb discrepancy in volume or circumference at point of most visible difference; obvious swelling or obscuration of anatomic architecture; obliteration of skin folds, readily apparent differences from anatomic contours

- Grade 3: more than 30% interlimb discrepancy in volume, lymphorrhea, gross deviation from normal anatomic contours, interferes with ADLs

- Grade 4: progression to malignancy (lymphangiosacroma), amputation indicated; disabling lymphedema

Conservative management techniques for lymphedema

- Elevation

- Compression wrapping

- Manual lymph drainage massage techniques

- Low resistance exercise of distal musculature

- Upper limb exercises do not increase risk of onset of lymphedema post breast cancer therapy

- Extreme exercise may promote inflammation and injuries, and should be avoided in those at risk of lympdedema

- Progressive, titrated exercises are helpful; start at low intensity, progress slowly and according to symptom response

Cancer pain

- May be due to many conditions, both tumour process-related and treatment-related

- Common treatment related pains include mucositis, peripheral neuropathy

- Common malignant cause of pain may include tumour invasion of bone from metastasis, compression/infiltration of peripheral nerves

- WHO recommends stepwise use of non-opioid analgesics, adjuvant drugs, and opioids, matching severity of pain to appropriate potency analgesics

- Aspirin and NSAIDS are useful for pain associated with bone metastases as they are potent prostaglandins synthetase inhibitors, but therapeutic ceiling prevents significant dose escalation

- Corticosteroids prevent release of prostaglandins and are helpful to reduce pain associated with tumour infiltration of viscera, bone, peripheral nerves and spinal cord

- Adjuvant therapies may include tricyclics antidepressants, anti-epileptics, duloxetine

- Opioids have no ceiling effects, though side effects may necessitate changes in routes of administration or rotation to other agents

- Invasive pain management may be indicated if

  - pain becomes intractable and not relieved by increasing dosages of opioids or rotation to another opiate

  - pain medications lead to overwhelming and unmanageable side effects

  - pain responds poorly to opioid therapy and intra-axial (intrathecal) delivery may be beneficial. Other options include neurolytic blocks, spinal administration, and surgical neuro-ablative procedures

11

Adult Joint Reconstruction Rehabilitation

LUI Wen Li, KIM Jongmoon

Hip osteoarthritis (OA)

- 3–8 times body weight are exerted on the hip joint during weight-bearing activities (walking, running, jumping, lifting)

- Risk factors: aging, hip trauma (unilateral), obesity (bilateral), occupational heavy lifting, frequent stair climbing

- Primary hip OA (most common) vs. secondary (prior hip trauma, joint infection, congenital or other deformities)

- Symptoms: groin pain, hip joint stiffness, functional limitations

- Physical examination

  - Antalgic gait: limp with decreased single-limb stance time on painful limb, shortened stride length for contralateral limb, increased double support time

  - Decreased hip range of motion: loss of hip internal rotation is the earliest sign of hip OA

  - Patrick test or FABER (hip flexion, abduction, external rotation) manoeuvre

  - Hip abductor weakness (Trendelenburg gait)

- Differential diagnosis

  - Intra-articular: avascular necrosis, labral tear, joint infection, acetabular fracture, inflammatory arthropathy

  - Extra-articular: proximal femur fracture, bursitis (trochanteric, ischial, iliopsoas), iliotibial band tendinitis, piriformis or gluteal muscle strain or myofascial pain, snapping hip, lumbosacral radiculopathy, sacroiliac joint pain

- Conservative treatment
    - Medications: paracetamol, oral NSAIDs
    - Weight management
    - Exercise programme: range of motion, muscle strengthening (static → dynamic), aerobic conditioning by walking or aquatic therapy
    - Walking cane, correction of leg length discrepancy, adaptive equipment (reachers, sock donners, long-handled shoe horns)
    - Fluoroscopy or ultrasound guided hip joint intra-articular corticosteroid injections: improves pain and function for several months

Knee osteoarthritis

- Three major knee compartments: medial, lateral, patellofemoral
    - Medial compartment: most commonly involved, leading to genu varum (bow leg)
    - Lateral compartment: leading to genu valgum (knock-knee)
- Risk factors: age, obesity, sports injuries, vigorous physical activity, work-related activities (heavy physical work with knee bending, squatting, kneeling)
- Symptoms and signs: knee pain, stiffness, tenderness, decreased range of motion, crepitus, effusion
- Medications: paracetamol, NSAIDs (oral or topical), capsaicin cream, nutritional intervention (glucosamine, chondroitin)
- Intra-articular injection
    - Corticosteroid: short term relief of symptoms, reduction of local inflammation
    - Viscosupplementation (hyaluronic acid): protective properties to synovial fluid (shock absorption, energy dissipation, lubrication), less effective for pain relief but more prolonged effect than corticosteroid

Knee osteoarthritis rehabilitation

- Exercise: relieves pain, enhances functional capacity
  - Strengthening exercise (especially of quadriceps): improvements in strength, pain, function and quality of life
  - Aerobic exercise (exercise bicycle, walking): alleviates pain and joint tenderness, promotes functional status and respiratory capacity, positive effects on mood and motivation
- Therapeutic modalities: Transcutaneous Electrical Nerve Stimulation (TENS), massage, stretching (hamstring, quadriceps), heat (for chronic pain), cold (for acute pain)
- Adaptive equipment: cane or walker (reduces hip or knee loading, reduces pain, prevents falls)
- Bracing and footwear: knee brace, lateral heel wedge (lessens medial load across the knee), patellar taping or brace (realign patella), correction of leg length discrepancy
- Acupuncture
- Weight management: if BMI ≥ 25
- Arthritis Self Management Program (ASMP)

Arthritis self management program (ASMP)

- Patient education program
- 6 weeks interactive workshop (2 hours, once a week)
  - Techniques to deal with problems such as pain, fatigue, frustration and isolation
  - Appropriate exercise for maintaining and improving strength, flexibility, and endurance
  - Appropriate use of medications
  - Communicating effectively with family, friends, and health professionals
  - Healthy eating
  - Making informed treatment decisions
  - Disease-related problem solving
  - Getting a good night's sleep

Osteoarthritis Research International (OARSI) guidelines for non-surgical management of knee OA

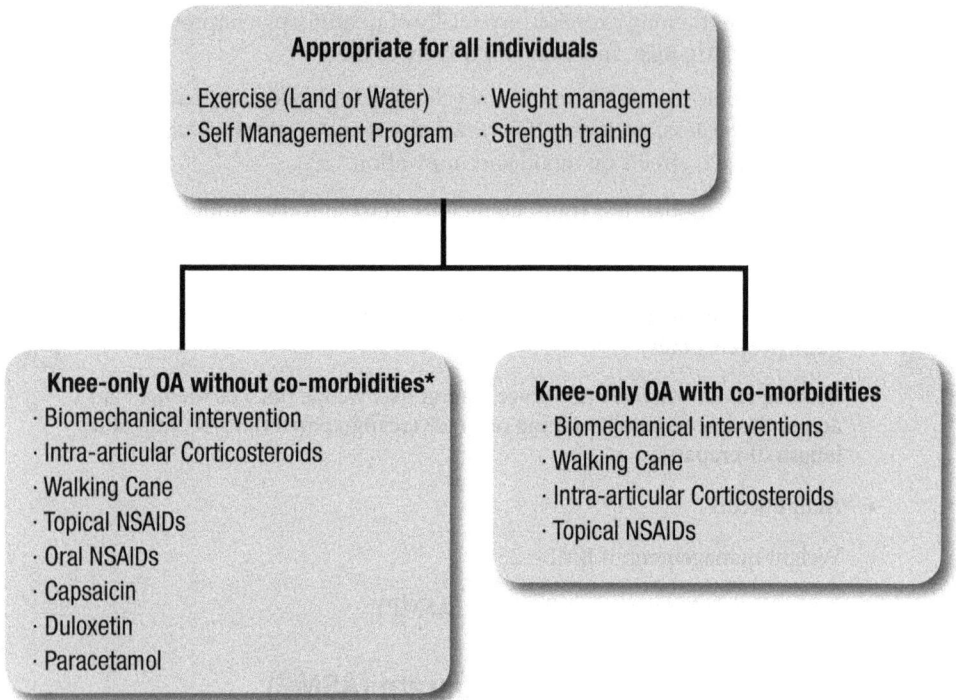

Appropriate for all individuals

· Exercise (Land or Water) · Weight management
· Self Management Program · Strength training

Knee-only OA without co-morbidities*
· Biomechanical intervention
· Intra-articular Corticosteroids
· Walking Cane
· Topical NSAIDs
· Oral NSAIDs
· Capsaicin
· Duloxetin
· Paracetamol

Knee-only OA with co-morbidities
· Biomechanical interventions
· Walking Cane
· Intra-articular Corticosteroids
· Topical NSAIDs

*Co-morbidities: diabetes, hypertension, cardiovascular disease, renal failure, gastrointestinal bleeding, depression, physical impairment limiting activity (including obesity)

Hip fractures

- Types of hip fractures (classified by anatomic location and fracture type)
    - Intracapsular (femoral neck and head of femur)
    - Extracapsular (intertrochanteric and subtrochanteric)
- Symptoms: hip pain and swelling, bruising around the hip, inability to bear weight
- Physical examination
    - Ecchymosis around the hip (especially extracapsular fractures)
    - Shortened and externally rotated lower limb
    - Tenderness over the trochanteric area

- ▪ Assess for other injuries (all other extremities and spine)
- Investigations
    - ▪ AP pelvis radiograph (to compare with the uninvolved hip) and lateral radiograph of the hip
    - ▪ MRI hip (if plain radiographs are unrevealing but a fracture is suspected clinically)
- Complications
    - ▪ Increased risk of mortality and morbidity in both short term (3–6 months) and long term (5–10 years)
    - ▪ Blood loss from fracture (especially extracapsular fractures)
    - ▪ Infections
    - ▪ Thromboembolism
    - ▪ Delirium
- Management
    - ▪ Evaluate reason for fall (e.g. syncope, stroke)
    - ▪ Assess for concomitant injuries
    - ▪ Adequate analgesia
    - ▪ Thromboembolism prophylaxis
        - ◆ Early mobilisation
        - ◆ Pneumatic leg compression
        - ◆ Low molecular weight heparin is recommended (at least 12 hours pre-operatively to 10–14 days post operatively and until the patient is fully ambulatory)
- Definitive management
    - ▪ Non-surgical treatment (in severely debilitated patients) — will be at best wheelchair bound
    - ▪ Surgical treatment
        - ◆ Should be performed within 48 hours of hospitalization and not be delayed for more than 72 hours
        - ◆ Neck of femur fractures: cancellous screws vs bipolar hemiarthroplasty

- Intertrochanteric fractures: proximal femoral nail anti-rotation
- Prevention and management of delirium
  - Avoid factors known to cause or worsen delirium: physical restraints, urinary catheters, infections, drug use, fluid/electrolyte disturbances, pain
  - Identify and treat the underlying acute illness
  - Provide supportive and restorative care to prevent further physical and cognitive decline
  - Control dangerous and disruptive behaviours so the first three steps can be accomplished
- Assessment for underlying osteoporosis
  - Should be treated with bisphosphonate
  - Baseline Bone Mineral Densitometry (BMD)
- Fall prevention

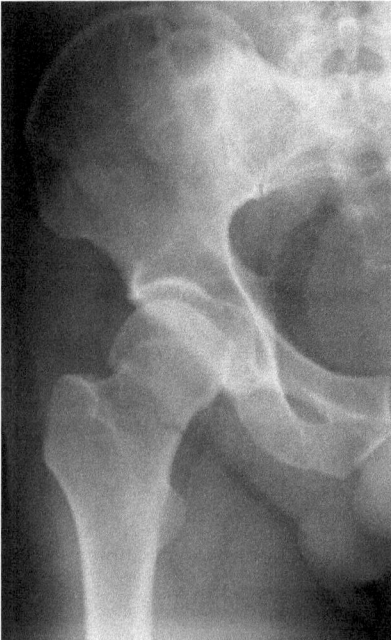

Fig. 1. Neck of femur fracture.

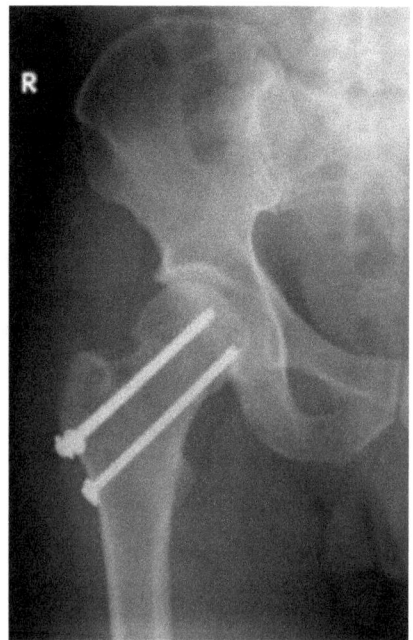

Fig. 2. Cancellous screws.

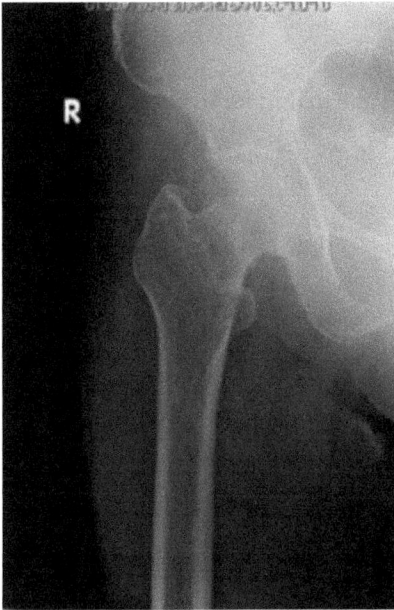

Fig. 3. Neck of femur fracture.

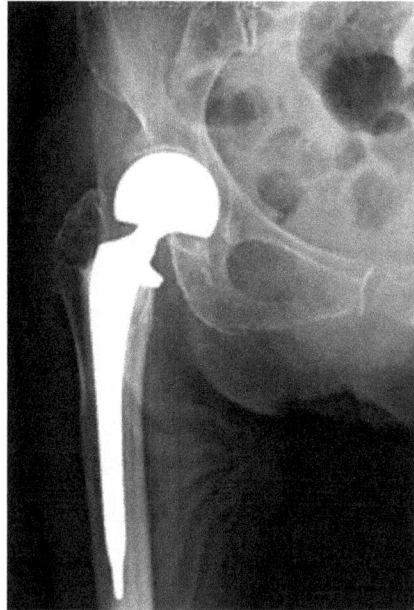

Fig. 4. Bipolar hemiarthroplasty.

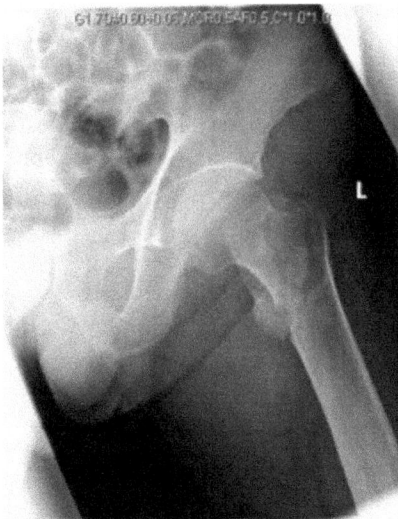

Fig. 5. Intertrochanteric fracture.

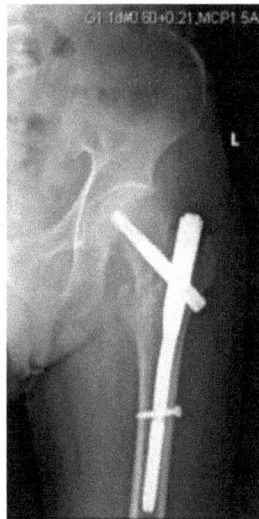

Fig. 6. Proximal femoral nail antirotation.

Osteoporosis

- Hip fracture is a manifestation of severe osteoporosis, hence patients with a recent hip fracture should be evaluated and treated for osteoporosis

- Hip fractures are followed by a 2.5-fold increased risk of future fractures

- Investigations

  - BMD: to establish a baseline to monitor treatment response, but not to determine whether to initiate treatment

  - Investigations to rule out secondary causes of osteoporosis if indicated

- Management

  - Calcium and vitamin D supplementation if required

  - Replete vitamin D

  - Pharmacological intervention for osteoporosis is indicated for patient with fragility fractures, regardless of bone density findings

  - Bisphosphonates are considered first line drugs

Total hip arthroplasty (THA)

- Prosthetic replacement of the proximal femur and acetabulum

- Indications: osteoarthritis, inflammatory arthritis, avascular necrosis, post-traumatic degenerative joint disease, congenital hip disease, oncologic bone disease, infection

- Cemented vs. biologic or "press-fit" integration

- Anterior vs. anterolateral vs. direct lateral vs. posterior (posterolateral) approaches

- Hemiarthroplasty

  - Replacement of the proximal femur only

  - Reserved for patients with a healthy articular surface in the acetabulum

  - Most commonly seen after proximal femur fractures

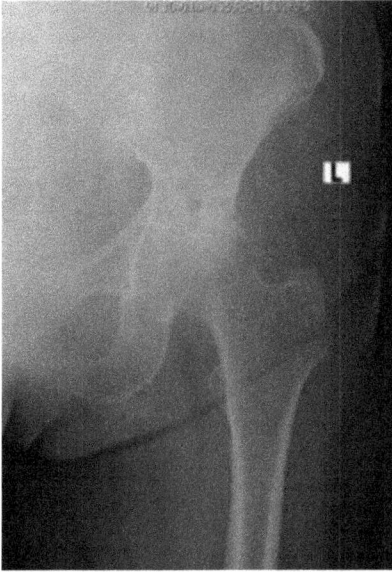

Fig. 7. Hip osteoarthritis and avascular necrosis.

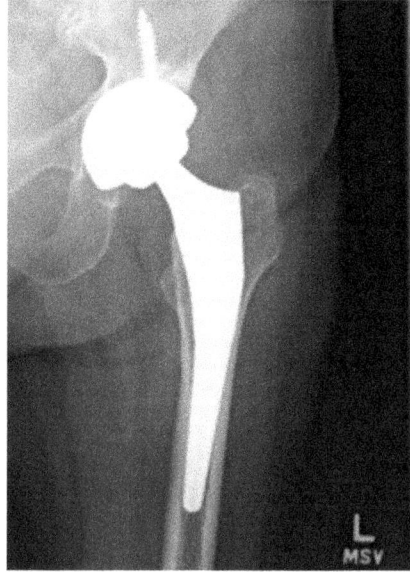

Fig. 8. Total hip arthroplasty (uncemented).

Total knee arthroplasty (TKA)

- Prosthetic replacement of the knee joint: resection of abnormal articular surfaces of the knee with resurfacing with metal and polyethylene components

- Indications: osteoarthritis (idiopathic or traumatic), inflammatory arthritis, avascular necrosis, tumor, congenital abnormalities

- Technique

  - Anterior approach (medial parapatellar approach): most common

  - Removal of osteophytes and intra-articular soft tissues

  - Femur and tibia end cut perpendicular to mechanical axis

  - Release ligaments and resurface patellofemoral joint if necessary

  - Placement of implants (cemented or press-fit)

- Immediate postoperative care

  - Adequate hydration

  - Adequate analgesia: continuation of intraoperative epidural, patient-controlled intravenous analgesia, or oral analgesia

  - Cryotherapy, range of motion (ROM) exercises or continuous passive motion (CPM)

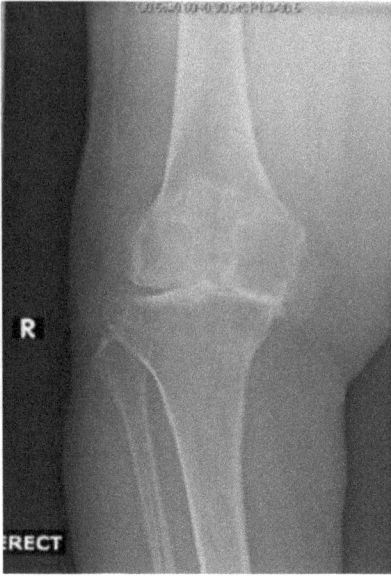

Fig. 9. Knee osteoarthritis.

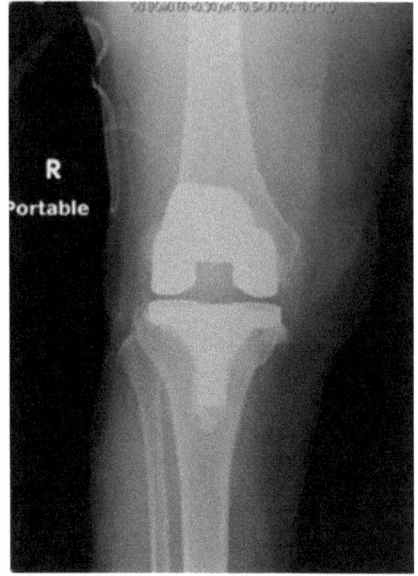

Fig. 10. Total knee arthroplasty.

Complications of total joint replacement

1. Aseptic loosening

- Pathology
    - Periprosthetic osteolysis
    - Wear debris generated from the implant stimulates inflammatory cells to promote bone resorption
- Symptoms: pain in the groin or buttocks after THA or about the knee after TKA
- Radiographic features
    - Peri-implant lucency
    - Progressive and extensive widening of interfaces between bone-cement, bone-prosthesis, or cement-prosthesis
    - Movement or fracture of the component
- Treatment: revision arthroplasty if severe pain and disability

2. Thromboembolic disease (deep venous thrombosis, DVT)

- The leading cause of death after total joint replacement
- Incidence of DVT
  - After THA: 40–60% in Western countries, 8–9.7% in Singapore
  - After TKA: 46–84% in Western countries, 14–22% in Singapore
- Manifestation: pain, swelling, warmth, tenderness, Homan's sign
- Diagnosis
  - D-dimer: to rule out DVT, not to confirm the diagnosis of DVT (high sensitivity 97%, poor specificity 35%)
  - Duplex ultrasonography (first-line imaging examination)
  - Impedance plethysmography
  - Venography

DVT prophylaxis

- Mechanical prophylaxis
  - Limb elevation, early mobilization, compression stocking
  - Intermittent pneumatic compression
  - Continuous passive motion
- Pharmacological prophylaxis
  - Low-molecular-weight heparin
  - direct thrombin inhibitors, direct factor Xa inhibitors
- Duration of pharmacological prophylaxis
  - Minimum of 10 to 14 days, up to 35 days (American College of Chest Physicians recommendation in 2012)
  - Adequate mobilisation is achieved

3. Infection

- Stage I: acute postoperative
  - Superficial (minimal drainage, pain, or erythema): IV or oral antibiotics, aggressive local dressing changes

- Deep (persistent drainage, leukocytosis, fever): irrigation, debridement, arthrotomy, excision
- Stage II: deep delayed
  - Painful joint, there may be absence of other clinical findings with normal erythrocyte sedimentation rate (ESR)
  - Treatment: excision of the arthroplasty, placement of cement spacer, revision arthroplasty after adequate IV antibiotics
- Stage III: late
  - Hematogenous spread during dental procedure or urinary tract infection (UTI)
  - Joint pain and dysfunction, elevated ESR
  - Treatment: excision of the arthroplasty, placement of cement spacer, revision arthroplasty after adequate IV antibiotics

Antibiotic prophylaxis for patients after total joint replacement

- Information statement from the AAOS (American Academy of Orthopaedic Surgeons) in 2009
- Consider antibiotic prophylaxis for all total joint replacement patients prior to any invasive procedure that may cause bacteremia
- Patients at potential increased risk of hematogenous total joint infection
  - All patients with prosthetic joint replacement
  - Immunocompromised/immunosuppressed patients
  - Inflammatory arthropathies
  - Patients with co-morbidities: diabetes, obesity, HIV, smoking, hemophilia, malnourishment
  - Previous prosthetic joint infections
  - Megaprostheses

4. Heterotopic ossification

- Common after THA (as high as 80%), 3.8–32% after TKA
- Functionally significant ectopic bone is rare (< 10% of cases)

- High risk: men with hypertrophic OA, ankylosing spondylitis, or DISH syndrome and patients with a previous history of heterotopic bone

- Symptoms and signs: persistent pain, swelling, or warmth about the hip (after THA) or anterior thigh (after TKA) 2 or 3 weeks after surgery

- Diagnosis: persistently elevated alkaline phosphatase, radiographs (not positive until at least 3 weeks), bone scan, ultrasound

- Treatment: bisphosphonates, NSAIDs, excision (after maturation)

5. Peripheral nerve injuries

- Incidence: 1–2% after primary THA, 3–4% after revision THA, 1.3% after TKA

- Affected nerve

  - Sciatic nerve (peroneal division) > femoral nerve in THA

  - Peroneal nerve > tibial nerve in TKA

- Mechanism of injury: compressive forces, direct trauma, ischemia

- Prognosis: complete recovery 50% in THA, 68% in TKA

6. Hip dislocation

- Incidence

  - 0.2–10% after primary THA, 28% after revision THA

  - Posterior dislocation after a posterior approach: ¾ of all dislocation

  - > 50% within the first 4–6 weeks

- Risk factors

  - Surgical approach (posterior > anterior)

  - Prosthetic components size and orientation

  - Weakness of muscle and soft tissue supporting structures

  - Multiple revision surgeries

  - Non-adherence to ROM restrictions

  - Individual patient factors (cognitive impairment, female, old age)

- Manifestations: hip pain, limited range of motion, "pop" sound, leg in an abducted and internally rotated position in posterior dislocation

- Treatment

  ■ Closed reduction within the first few hours after dislocation

  ■ Surgical reduction for patients with failure of closed reduction, ≥ 2 dislocations, late dislocation (≥ 5 years)

Hip dislocation prevention

- Hip precautions

  ■ For patients with posterior approach to surgery

  ■ Up to 6–12 weeks following surgery

    ◆ Avoid hip flexion of more than 90°

    ◆ Avoid hip adduction past midline

    ◆ Avoid hip internal rotation past neutral

- Adaptive equipment: abduction pillow, raised toilet seat, long-handled reacher, long shoe horn, etc.

- Patient education: "Do not bend over too far, Do not lean over to get up, Do not sit low on a toilet or chair, Do not cross your legs, Do not stand with toes turned in, Do not lie on your side without a pillow between your legs, etc."

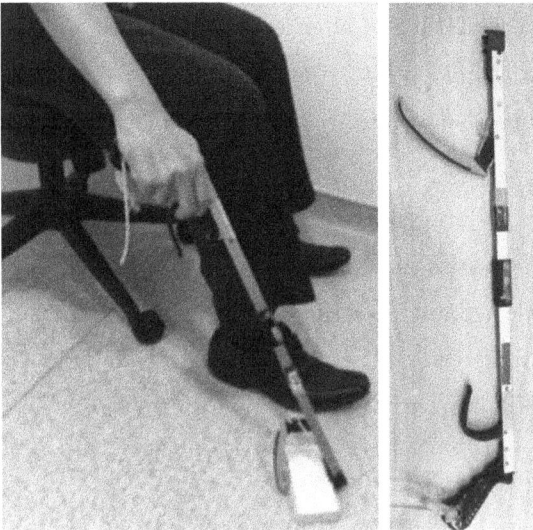

Fig. 11. Long-handled reacher.

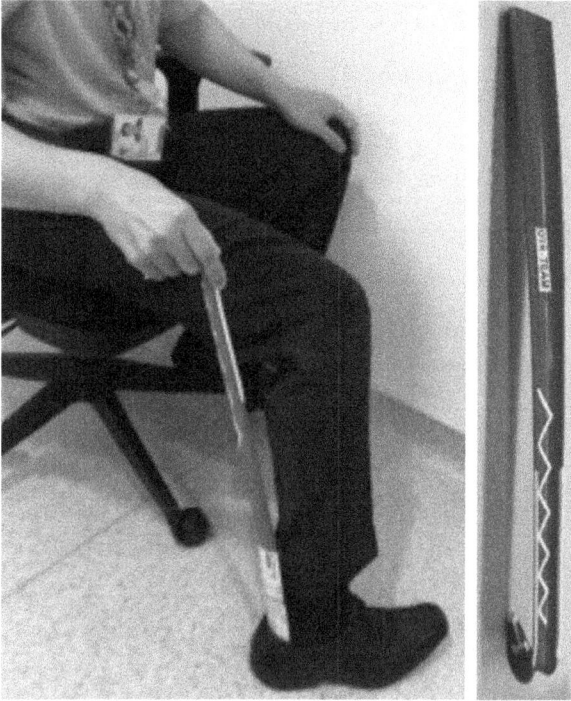

Fig. 12. Long shoe horn.

Goals of rehabilitation after THA

- Successful postoperative pain management
- Maintain medical stability
- Achieve successful surgical incision healing
- Guard against dislocation of the implant
- Prevent bed rest hazards
- Obtain pain-free range of motion within precaution limits
- Strengthen hip and knee musculature
- Gain functional strength
- Teach transfers and ambulation with assistive devices
- Successful progression to prior living situation

Goals of rehabilitation after TKA

- Successful postoperative pain management
- Maintain medical stability
- Achieve successful surgical incision healing
- Prevent bed rest hazards
- Obtain pain-free 0–90° of knee range of motion in the first 2 weeks
- Rapid return of quadriceps control and strength
- Safety during ambulation and transfers
- Successful progression to prior living situation

Total joint replacement rehabilitation program

Medical care

- Pain control
  - Administration of analgesics should be performed round the clock rather than just on an as needed (prn) basis
  - Controlled-release and short-acting opioids may be used
  - Causes of pain: operative site problem (infection, mechanical failure), nerve injury, vascular origin
- Bladder and bowel functions
  - Removal of indwelling catheter, check post-void residual urine volume
  - Causes of constipation: decreased mobility, post- anesthesia effect, narcotic analgesics
  - Adequate bowel program: stool softener, laxatives, enema
- Adequate nutrition and hydration
- Manage anemia due to blood loss during surgery

Muscle strengthening

- Isometric strengthening of quadriceps and hip extensors muscles should be started immediately after surgery

- Progressive resistive exercise, using the weight of the lower limb, straight-leg-raise (SLR) (hip flexion and knee extension) may be started within the first few days of surgery when partial weight bearing or full weight bearing is permitted: SLR applies a force of 1.5–1.8 times the body weight

- Resistance may be added as tolerated

- Initially, active hip abduction should be done in a supine position

- For TKA, additional resistance for SLR/knee extension should be avoided until full active extension is achieved (risk of quad tendon rupture)

- Overall muscle strengthening: upper extremity (for using assistive devices and transfers), non-operated limb (for ambulation and transfers)

Range-of-motion exercises (ROM)

- Full ROM at all non-operated joints: active ROM or passive ROM (several times a day)

- THA or hemiarthroplasty: specific hip ROM exercises are not indicated (hip precaution)

- TKA: knee flexion and extension exercise should begin as soon as possible after recovery from surgery

- Continuous passive motion (CPM) machine: up to 90°; controversial, may shorten hospital stay

- Required knee ROM in normal function

  - Stair climbing step over step: 83°

  - Walking in swing phase: 70°

  - Standing up from a chair: 93°

  - Standing up from a toilet: 105°

- Knee ROM goal on discharge from hospital: 0–90°

- Mean knee ROM in long-term follow-up: 110–115°

Continuous passive motion (CPM)

- The long-term effects of CPM on ROM, DVT, PE, and pain relief are controversial

- May shorten the period of hospitalisation: achieve 90° of flexion earlier

- May increase incidence of wound complications: transcutaneous oxygen tension of the skin near the incision decreases significantly after the knee is flexed more than 40°

- CPM rate of one cycle per minute, 4–6 hours, and maximum flexion limited to 40° for the first 3 days, CPM progression of 10° per day thereafter

- Maximum flexion up to 90°

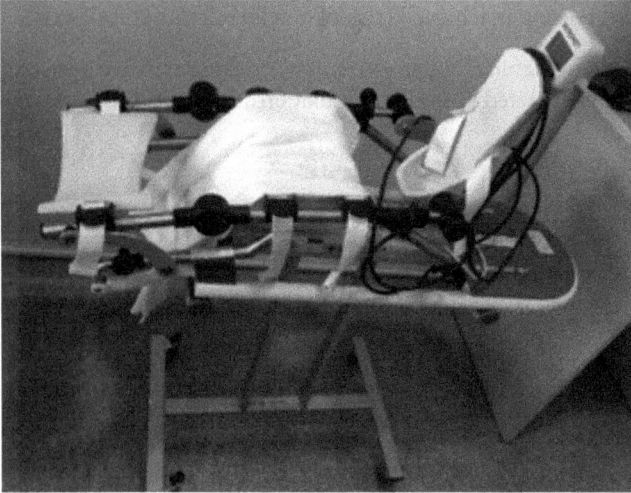

Fig. 13. CPM machine.

Weight-bearing principles

- Weight-bearing and activity restriction are influenced by surgical technique and surgeon preference

- Full weight bearing is generally allowed in cemented prosthesis and good press-fit implants

- Weight-bearing precautions
    - Non-weight-bearing (NWB)
    - Toe-touch weight-bearing (TTWB): up to 20% of body weight
    - Partial weight-bearing (PWB): 20–50% of body weight
    - Weight-bearing as tolerated (WBAT): 50–100% of body weight
    - Full weight-bearing (FWB): 100% of body weight

Table 1. An example of a THA postoperative rehabilitation protocol

Post-operative day (POD) 1	POD 2
- Bedside exercises (ankle pumps, quadriceps sets, hamstring sets, gluteal sets) - Bed mobility and transfer (bed to/from chair)	- Continue previous exercises - Supine hip ROM within allowed ranges - Hip abduction active assisted ROM to active ROM - Heel slides - Bridging - Gait training with assistive device - Transfer training
POD 3-4	**POD 5 – 4 weeks**
- Continue previous exercises - Sitting heel raised - Large arc quads - Progression of ambulation on level surface and stair - ADL training	- Strengthening exercises (side- lying hip abduction, standing hip flexion/extension/abduction, Thera-Band exercise) - Mini-squats - Forward step-up - Progression of ambulation distance - Progression of independence with ADL

Table 2. An example of a TKA postoperative rehabilitation protocol.

POD 1	POD 2
- Bedside exercises (ankle pumps, quadriceps sets, hamstring sets,gluteal sets) - Bed mobility and transfer (bed to/from chair)	- active ROM, active assisted ROM, terminal knee extension exercise - Continue previous exercises - Gait training with assistive device on level surfaces - Functional transfer training (sit to/from stand, toilet transfer, bed mobility)

POD 3–5	POD 6–4 weeks
- Progression of ROM and strengthening exercises - Progression of ambulation distance, stair training with assistive device - ADL training	- ROM exercises: exercise bike, active assisted ROM for knee flexion, knee extension stretch, patellar mobilization - Strengthening exercises (quad sets, SLR, side-lying hip abduction, hamstring curls, sitting knee extension) - Ice and compression for pain or swelling - Incision mobility: soft tissue mobilization - Progression of ambulation distance, stairs, ADL - Cardiovascular exercise: upper body ergometer, exercise bicycle

Driving and sports activities

- Driving assessment should be considered for patients after total joint replacement in right lower limb: braking reaction time is prolonged until 8 weeks after surgery

- Able to resume sports activities with low-impact sports: swimming, cycling, golf, walking

- High-impact sports (running, single tennis, racquetball, basketball, baseball, soccer) should be avoided: high risk of aseptic loosening

Outcome measures after total joint replacement

- Patient-reported measures

  - Short Form-36 Health Questionnaire (SF-36)/SF-12

  - Western Ontario and McMaster Universities Osteoarthritis Index (WOMAC)

  - Oxford Hip Score (OHS)/Hip Disability and Osteoarthritis Outcome Score (HOOS)

  - Oxford Knee Score (OKS)/Knee Injury and Osteoarthritis Outcome Score (KOOS)

  - Knee Outcome Survey-Activities of Daily Living Scale (KOS-ADLS)

- ■ Knee Society Clinical Rating System (KSS)
- Performance-based measures
  - ■ Timed Up and Go Test (TUG)
  - ■ Stair Climbing Test (SCT)
  - ■ Six Minute Walk Test (6MWT)

Recommended reading

- Frontera WR, Silver JK, Rizzo Jr TD. Chapter 55: Hip osteoarthritis (pp. 285–290), Chapter 61: Total hip replacement (pp. 312–319), Chapter 70: Knee osteoarthritis (pp. 361–368), Chapter 80: Total knee replacement (pp. 411–418). In: Essentials of Physical Medicine and Rehabilitation, 3rd ed. Saunders, Philadelphia, 2014.

- DeLisa JA. Chapter 66: Rehabilitation of total hip and total knee replacement. In: Rehabilitation Medicine: Principles and Practice, 3rd ed. LWW, 2010.

- Brotzman SB, Manske RC. Chapter 6: The arthritic lower extremity. In: Clinical Orthopaedic Rehabilitation: An Evidence-based Approach, 3rd ed. Elsevier Mosby, Philadelphia, 2011.

- Guyatt GH, et al. Antithrombotic therapy and prevention of thrombosis, 9th ed: American College of Chest Physicians evidence-based clinical practice guidelines. Chest 2012;141(2)(Suppl):7S–47S.

- Zappe B, et al. Long-term prognosis of nerve palsy after total hip arthroplasty: results of two-year-follow-ups and long-term results after a mean time of 8 years. Arch Orthop Trauma Surg 2014;134(10):1477–1482.

- McAlindon TE, et al. OARSI guidelines for the non-surgical management of knee osteoarthritis. Osteoarthritis and Cartilage 2014;22(3):363–388.

- NICE. Hip fracture: management. NICE clinical guideline 124. Available at https://www.nice.org.uk/guidance/cg124 [NICE guideline]. 2011. Accessed 1 March 2016.

- Ministry of Health, Singapore. Osteoporosis. MOH clinical practice guidelines. Available at https://www.moh.gov.sg/content/dam/moh_web/HPP/Doctors/cpg_medical/withdrawn/cpg_Osteoporosis.pdf. 2008. Accessed 1 March 2016.

- American Academy of Orthopaedic Surgeons. Management of hip fractures in the elderly. American Academy of Orthopaedic Surgeons Evidence-Based Clinical Practice Guideline. Available at http://www.aaos.org/Research/guidelines/HipFxGuideline.pdf. 2014. Accessed 1 March 2016.

- Foster KW. Hip fractures in adults. In: UpToDate, Post TW (Ed). Waltham, MA. 2015.

- Morrison RS, Siu AL. Medical consultation for patients with hip fracture. In: UpToDate, Post TW (Ed). Waltham, MA. 2015.

12
Rehabilitation in the Intensive Care Unit

NEO Jong Jong

Background and introduction

Improved care in the intensive care unit (ICU) has resulted in improved ICU survival. However, ICU survivors have to live with significant sequelae. An example is ICU acquired weakness, which is the diffuse, symmetric, generalized muscle weakness that develops after the onset of critical illness. Risk factors for ICU acquired weakness include systemic inflammatory response syndrome, hyperglycemia, and certain medications like neuromuscular blocking agents.

Is there a role for early rehabilitation in the ICU? Studies have shown that early rehabilitation in the ICU setting is feasible, safe and of benefit in critically ill patients. It has also been found to result in better functional outcomes. This chapter aims to highlight the role of rehabilitation and rehabilitative interventions in the ICU setting.

Common sequelae in ICU survivors

Some common findings in ICU survivors are:

- Muscle weakness (ICU acquired weakness)

- Fatigue

- Exercise limitation

- Depression

- Complications of immobility and pressure related neurological deficits

- Disabilities secondary to injuries (e.g. memory loss from head injury, physical disabilities from orthopedic injuries)

- Post traumatic stress disorder

- Lower than normal health-related quality of life

- Inability to return to work

Definition

Early rehabilitation in the ICU refers to early rehabilitation assessment, early physical therapy, occupational therapy and other rehabilitation activities initiated immediately upon achieving physiologic stability and continued throughout the ICU stay. It can start within days of initiation of mechanical ventilation. The patient may still require mechanical ventilation, vasopressors and dialysis.

Is it safe?

Physical and occupational therapy in the early days of critical illness was found to be safe and well tolerated, and resulted in better functional outcomes at hospital discharge, a shorter duration of delirium, and more ventilator-free days compared with standard care.

However, early rehabilitation in the ICU is not without risks, and we should be mindful of the potential safety issues like:

- Physiological responses associated with exertion
- Need for alteration in medical plan of care, sedatives, or vasopressor administration
- Line dislodgement
- Accidental extubation

In a systemic review, the overall occurrence of the above events was found to be less than 4% of all patient interactions and none were deemed serious.

Is it good?

Examples of positive outcomes:

- Functional mobility
- Quality of life
- Length of stay, duration of mechanical ventilation and cost savings

Goals of early rehabilitation assessment

- Diagnosis and medical management of conditions causing complex disabilities
- Anticipation and prevention of physical, psychological and social complications, based on natural history and prognosis of diagnoses

- Identify specific areas for early rehabilitation intervention

- Evaluation of potential to gain from rehabilitation and prognosis for recovery

- Defining rehabilitation needs/goals and directing patients to appropriate rehabilitation services

- Collaborating and coordinating care with ICU team, other medical and therapy teams

- Communicating with families to provide relevant information, support them in distress and manage expectations

Principles of rehabilitation assessment

Global assessment

- Review of medical and surgical history

- Review of previous functional status

- Mental status/alertness

- Cardiac status

- Pulmonary status

- Neurological status

- Musculoskeletal status

- Skin integrity/edema

- Medications

- Presence of multiple tubes/drains/monitoring devices/orthopaedic devices/splints

Specific assessment

- Functional status including means of communication and vision

- Pain issues

- Agitation and its likely causes, e.g. pain, discomfort

- Identify early physical therapy goals

- Actively identify potential areas of intervention, e.g. prevention of contractures (e.g. splinting), presence of pain (analgesics), cognitive reorientation

Potential areas of rehabilitation interventions

- Sleep deprivation and over-sedation
- Pain
- Nutritional support/supplements
- Bowel care
- Prevention of deep vein thrombosis and prophylaxis
- Immobility and wasting
- Speech, communication
- Alertness and orientation
- Team communication with family
- Coordination of medical and ancillary disciplines
- Psychosocial issues and quality of life
- Caregiver stress

Goals of early physical therapy in ICU

Goals of physiotherapy

- Achieve early and progressive upright posture (verticalisation)
- Prevent or attenuate neuromuscular complications arising from immobility and prolonged bed rest
- Early functional mobility
- Specific muscle training
- Prevention of contractures
- Prevention of pressure-related nerve and soft tissue injuries

Goals of occupational therapy

- Achieve early upright/seated posture for functional activities of daily living
- Sensory/basal stimulation (e.g. acquired brain injury patient)
- Orientation, enhancing alertness with functional upper limb tasks

- Oedema management
- Maintenance of muscle and soft tissue length (limb position, usage of resting upper limb splints)
- Early seated activities of daily living (ADL) training (combing, wiping hands/face, wiping table — modified closed chain exercise)

When to mobilise?

- Patient selection protocol (may be ICU-specific: surgical, medical, cardio, neuro)
- Mental status (Richmond Agitation Sedation Scale, +1 to -1)
- Cardiovascular status (no recent arrhythmias, no inotrope/vasopressor infusions)
- Respiratory status (e.g. FiO2 < 50%, PEEP < 8)
- Titrate activities according to patient triage and alertness and cooperativeness

When not to mobilise?

- Excessive changes in cardiopulmonary parameters like heart rate, blood pressure, and respiratory rate
- Worsening alertness/increased agitation
- Worsening biochemical/hematological profiles

How to progress?

Tolerated pre-walking activities including:

- Bed mobility, sitting over edge of bed, sit to stand, full standing posture, weight shifting on legs
- Stable neurological, hemodynamics and cardiopulmonary status maintained

Assistive equipment

- Splints
- Pressure garment

- Pressure relief cushion
- Geriatric chair
- High backed wheelchair
- Recliner wheelchair
- Tilt-in-space wheelchair
- Modified call bell
- Modified high wheeled walker/platform rollator
- Bed that can be converted to upright chair configuration (e.g. Hill Rom)
- Inflation-exflation machine (e.g. CoughAssist)

Technology may facilitate rehabilitation in patients who cannot actively participate in therapy during the acute phase of their illness. Examples of rehabilitation therapeutics and technology used in relatively novel setting include:

- Neuromuscular electrical stimulation
- Cycle ergometry
- Motomed

Rehabilitation team

- ICU physician
- Rehabilitation physician
- Therapists (PT, OT, RT)
- Nurses
- Dietician
- Medical social worker

Other important medical/surgical professionals in the ICU

The planning and progression of mobilisation is also done in consultation with other surgical professionals like the orthopaedic surgeons, trauma surgeons and neurosurgeons. With early clearance for weight bearing status from the orthopaedics, a patient can progress in his rehabilitation without delay. Multitrauma patients have challenging issues including open abdomen, high intra-abdominal pressure or open wounds that need to be addressed before mobilisation. As for head injured patients, before starting rehabilitation interventions, issues of high intracranial pressures and need for further neurosurgical intervention should be addressed and anticipated.

When the ICU patient is assessed to have a grave prognosis, the palliative care physician steps in, minimising patient suffering, and communicating and supporting the patient's family.

Summary

Rehabilitation is not only about mobilisation; it is also about optimising a patient for mobilisation. The acute status of the ICU patient poses various problems to treating therapists. It challenges them to customise care and problem solve using strategies that suit both the patient and his/her unique enivronment. Co-ordinating physical therapy sessions with sedative interruption may enable early rehabilitation. Overcoming these barriers will require changing the ICU culture to one that prioritises early rehabilitation through interdisciplinary coordination, communication, and teamwork. It involves a well co-ordinated team (medical, surgical, nursing, allied health professionals) working to optimise the patient overall for the purpose of mobilisation and working towards increasing functional ability.

Recommended reading

- Schweickert WD, et al. Early physical and occupational therapy in mechanically ventilated, critically ill patients: a randomised controlled trial. Lancet 2009;373(9678):1874–1882.

- Adler J, Malone D. Early mobilisation in the ICU: a systemic review. *Cardiopulm Phys Ther J* 2012;23(1):5–13.

13

Pain in the Rehabilitation Patient Population: A Systems Approach

CHAN Kay Fei

'To cure sometimes, to relieve often, and to comfort always.'
Ascribed to Hippocrates

Ten reasons why optimal pain management is important

1. Pain is prevalent in the general and specific rehabilitation population. The prevalence of pain in the general rehabilitation population is up to 21%, in the stroke population 32% to 47%, and in the spinal cord injury population, as high as 81% at 1 year and 85% at 25 years

2. Can be persistent beyond acute injury, e.g. phantom pain, complex regional pain syndromes

3. Affects functional independence in older adults out in the community

4. Prevents participation in therapy and other activities

5. Affects mood and sleep and lowers quality of life, including sexual activities

6. Can be iatrogenic—urinary catheterisation and dressing change, post-therapy muscle pain and overuse syndromes, improper handling of subluxed hemiplegic shoulders

7. Pain is a signal for missed diagnosis which may manifest in the rehabilitation setting

    -   When patient emerges from coma; missed visceral injuries and neuropathies in acute stabilisation settings

    -   Evolving "red flags" related to backache, poor fitting of orthoses, prostheses and medical equipment, impending breakdown of skin integrity

8. Aggressive medications may lead to problems of polypharmacy, addictions and drug-drug interactions including drowsiness, gait unsteadiness and falls.

Neuroleptic malignant syndrome as a special rare syndrome for recognition and prompt treatments

9. Organised team approach well-placed for a biopsychosocial approach to chronic and persistent pain and its attendant problems of reduced activity, disturbed sleep and mood

10. Finally, pain is found in healthcare workers themselves from workplace musculoskeletal disorders (WMSD). Occupational backache may be as high as 45 to 60% of staff population

Ten keys to a good pain assessment

1. Obtain a good pain history: Where is it painful, when and how long (at rest, movement, night), What is it like (pain descriptors, e.g. tingling, dull aches, etc.), Whither (radiating patterns and dermatomal, mesodermal radiating patterns), exacerbating and relieving factors, pain phenomena—hyperalgesia, allodynia, etc.

2. Pain severity: pain scores, Wong–Baker "faces", descriptors, other pain scales

3. Associations: negative symptoms (numbness/weakness), colour, temperature and sudomotor changes (e.g. Complex Regional Pain Syndrome)

4. Functional and mood disturbances: activity limitations (work, hobbies, endurance, work hours), sleep disturbances, depression or anxiety

5. Complete inventory of medications, modalities, procedures, radiological/neurophysiological evaluations, psychotherapy and complementary interventions received and benefits/adverse effects. Note drug allergies

6. Recognise special situations like drug dependence, doctor hopping, attention-seeking behaviour, conversion disorders and even malingering (difficult to conclusively prove) behaviours, return to work difficulties, pain in vulnerable populations—elderly, young, non-communicative, cognitively impaired

7. Examine the affected painful area carefully and systematically—exclude urgent (neuro)surgical events and visceral pathologies. Pay special attention to trauma and surgical sites (look for wound infection, infected implants, instability and fracture of implants, stump neuroma). For musculoskeletal pain, look for active movements before passive movements, kinetic chain considerations/disordered biomechanics, tenderness and myofascial trigger points, musculoskeletal and neurological examinations, observe for skin breaks, skin colour changes, surface temperature change, inflamed joints (inflammatory arthritis vs. heterotopic ossification) and abnormal hair growth

8. Observe the gait, facial expressions and activities of patient in multiple settings. Feedback from caregivers for concordance and consistency of reported symptoms

9. Psychological and social assessments—for cognition assessments, loss of self-esteem, coping, suicidal ideations, post-traumatic stress disorders, relationship difficulties, doctor hopping

10. Assess the supporting networks of the patients like significant others, family and social circles and obtain independent observations of patient's pain behaviours and mood

Ten prescriptions for the rehabilitation team to better serve our patients with pain

1. Interdisciplinary and trans-disciplinary approach means that the well trained team owns the problem of pain, the 5th vital sign

2. Team observation allows us to observe the patient in pain over an extended period of time and see the response to pain interventions including for drug withdrawal syndromes

3. Pain management by the rehabilitation team extends beyond medications, modalities, muscle conditioning and special skills (e.g. manipulative therapy, needling, medical acupuncture, joint and nerve injections, botulinum toxin injections); special diagnostics (like diagnostic musculoskeletal ultrasound and neurophysiological tests) are domain speciality skills in a comprehensive rehabilitation centre

4. Additional interventions which optimise pain control through good inter-disciplinary practice should be explored

5. Good fitting orthotics for subluxed joints, pressure relief and prevention of contractures and maintenance of good posture. Good ergonomics of fitting the activity to the patient and healthcare worker

6. Timing of pain pharmacology before activity and for post-therapy pain

7. Return to work prescription, work hardening and work process change. Further injury prevention. Pain related fatigue and energy conservation should be examined

8. Liaison and advocacy: case management approach to patients with complex issues, family and employer conferences

9. Distraction, relaxation, stress management techniques

10. Quality of life issues: fitness, sexuality, hobbies, support groups

Ten important footnotes for the practising rehabilitation professional

1. Recognise the pain crisis: monitor a patient in severe pain often and closely. If there is severe and uncontrolled pain, refer urgently to the pain specialists in acute pain service or pain management centre

2. The agitated pain patient can be in pain crisis or have drug related adverse effects like serotonin syndrome (vs. neuroleptic malignant syndrome vs. central dysautonomia). Besides agitation and positive medication use, there could be cardiovascular instability, muscle tremors with or without fever in the latter conditions

3. Respect headaches in neurosurgical patients (raised intracranial pressure); high spinal cord injury patients (autonomic dysreflexia with relative hypertension) and analgesia-associated headache (especially in patients with analgesia cocktails)

4. There is increasing formal accreditation and accountability from practitioners for the prescriptive use of opioids in healthcare institutions. Check approved local practice

5. Advanced pain interventions: radiologically-guided nerve and deep joint injections, implantable pumps (of opioids and baclofen) and neuromodulation at the spinal cord and brain. The safe practice, monitoring of function and titration of management needs well-trained specialists, special equipment and special set-ups

6. Acupuncture and manual medicine/chiropractic practice/osteopathic practice: may be useful for acute musculoskeletal pain in well trained hands. Caution for excessive force upon poor bone integrity (osteoporosis and occult fractures), lax joints and tight spinal canals can potentially lead to severe (iatrogenic) neurological injuries from treatments

7. Pain is still a subjective complaint and the word of the patient is best taken seriously at the clinical encounter. Trust between patient and doctor/healthcare provider should be established as a priority especially for chronic pain patients

8. The hospital is an ecosystem to manage pain beyond the rehabilitation settings. Other pain practitioners/specialists are found in the pain

management centre, acute pain service, palliative medicine service and geriatric pain services, etc. Rehabilitation physicians contribute to the chronic pain clinics and manage musculoskeletal pain syndromes like backache, recreational sports injuries and fibromyalgia

9. Neuroplasticity and pain: mechanisms which relate to pain potentiation, modulation and amplification is beyond the scope of our discussions here. The interested reader is directed elsewhere to understand better the enlarging and emerging field

10. We will see the ravages of loss of pain and other sensory modalities in insensate limbs like recalcitrant ulcers, limb loss and neuropathic joints. These sensory inputs are protective in themselves. However, it is the disease conditions of chronic and persistent pain with wide-ranging biological debilitating effects, psychosocial impact and loss of function and quality of life that our strenuous attention and efforts are directed against

Recommended reading

- Walsh NE, Maria DS, Eckman M, 2010. Treatment of patients with chronic pain. In: Frontera WR. Delisa's Physical Medicine & Rehabilitation, 5th Edition. Lippincott Williams & Wilkins, pp 1273-1318.

- Treister AK, Hatch MN, Cramer SC, Chang EY. Demystifying Poststroke Pain: From Etiology to Treatment. PM R. 2016 Jun 16. pii: S1934-1482(16)30182-4

14
Practical Approach to Spasticity

SETIOTA Nuez Odessa, KONG Keng He

Definition

Lance (1980) defined spasticity as a motor disorder characterized by a velocity-dependent increase in the tonic stretch reflexes (muscle tone) with exaggerated tendon jerks resulting from hyper-excitability of the stretch reflex as one component of the upper motor neuron syndrome.

There are 2 components contributing to muscle tone:

1. Neural component—reflex activity

2. Non-neural components—rheological properties intrinsic to muscle and other soft tissues caused by inertia, elasticity and viscosity of the muscle that is moved

The following description by Peter Nathan (1973) nicely summarizes spasticity: "Spasticity is a condition in which stretch reflexes that are normally latent become obvious. In spasticity, the tendon reflexes have a lowered threshold to tap, the response of the tapped muscles is increased, and additional muscles besides the tapped one respond; tonic stretch reflexes are affected in the same way".

Causes of spasticity

Spasticity can be seen in upper motor neuron lesions and these include stroke, traumatic brain injury, spinal cord lesions, e.g. multiple sclerosis, suprasacral spinal cord injury and cerebral palsy.

Spasticity normally develops over a period of time after the upper motor neuron lesion, and although the exact mechanisms have yet to be fully elucidated, it is likely that reduction in spinal inhibitory mechanisms are involved.

Clinical signs of spasticity

As part of the upper motor neuron syndrome, spasticity can be associated with other positive and negative signs.

Positive signs include:

- Exaggerated tendon reflexes

- Enhanced primitive reflexes

- Spastic co-contraction: this refers to inappropriate simultaneous co-contraction of both agonist and antagonist muscles. For example, elbow extension in a stroke patient may appear weaker than it actually is because of co-contraction of the elbow flexors

- Associated reactions: this refers to involuntary movement of the affected body part when the unaffected body part is moved. An example is involuntary elbow flexion in stroke patients as they attempt to stand or walk

- Spasms: these could be extensor or flexor

- Clonus: this refers to involuntary, rhythmic, muscular contractions and relaxations due to a self-re-excitation of the hyperactive stretch reflexes in the affected muscle. An example is ankle clonus

  Negative signs include:

- Muscle weakness

- Loss of selective motor control with slowness of movements and decreased dexterity

- Fatigue due to greater effort expended in performing a motor task

Complications of spasticity

These include:

- Contractures

  - A spastic muscle is in a state of constant contraction, and this causes muscle shortening and increases the risk of muscle and joint contractures

- Pain

- Impaired passive function

- Examples include difficulty wearing of splints, difficulty with proper positioning in seating/lying, difficulty with perineal hygiene or toileting because of severe hip adductor spasticity

• Impaired active function

- Examples include gait difficulty because of excessive ankle plantarflexion and invertor spasticity; difficulty with upper limb forward reach because of elbow spasticity

• Altered body image

Table 1. Common spasticity patterns.

Common patterns	Muscles involved	Complications/side effects
Adducted/internally rotated shoulder	Pectoralis major, teres major, latissimus dorsi, subscapularis	• Shoulder pain on ranging • Difficulties in dressing, limitation in reaching forward
Flexed elbow	Biceps brachii, brachialis, brachioradialis	• Difficulties in transfer (no fulcrum), dressing and reaching • Stretch injury to the ulnar nerve (at the bend of the elbow). The nerve is vulnerable to repeated trauma and can be compressed in the cubital tunnel
Pronated forearm	Pronator teres, pronator quadratus	• Pain on supination
Flexed wrist	Flexor carpi radialis, flexor carpi ulnaris palmaris longus	• Compression of the median nerve at wrist with carpal tunnel syndrome • Weakened grip strength

Clenched fist	Flexor digitorum superficialis, flexor digitorum profundus	• Issues with hand hygiene • Difficulties with wearing of hand splints. Limitation of grasping, manipulation and release of objects
Thumb-in-palm deformity	• Flexor pollicis longus and brevis • Adductor pollicis, first dorsal interosseous	• Difficulty to execute grasp patterns (three-jaw chuck, lateral grasp and tip pinch)
Flexed hip	Iliopsoas and rectus femoris	• Interferes with positioning in chair • Walking with a crouched gait pattern and compensatory knee flexion to maintain balance (leading to fatigability)
Adducted thigh	Adductor longus, magnus and brevis	• Scissoring thighs interfere with perineal care, sexual intimacy, sitting, transfers,standing and walking • Difficulties with limb clearance and advancement during swing phase of gait
Stiff knee	Rectus femoris,vastus intermedius, medialis and lateralis	• Gait deviation with the knee remaining extended through the gait cycle • Functional lengthening of the leg during the gait with dragging of the toe and risk to trip and fall

Flexed knee	Medial and lateral hamstrings	• Compensation of ipsilateral hip flexion during stance phase with flexed knee and contralateral hip and knee flexion (crouch gait pattern)
		• Difficulties with transfers and wheelchair positioning
		• Limitation of limb advancement due to the lack of knee extension during terminal swing (short step length)
Equinovarus foot	• Medial and lateral gastrocnemius	• Skin breakdown on lateral border of foot
	• Soleus	• Pain upon weight bearing over the lateral border of the foot
	• Tibialis posterior and sometimes, tibialis anterior	• Difficulties with shoewear
	• Flexor digitorum longus	• Limitation of dorsiflexion during early and mid-stance with impaired ground clearance

Assessment of spasticity

Measures of impairment

Modified Ashworth Scale (MAS)

MAS is useful in clinical practice due to its ease and speed of use and widely used in research. It measures resistance to passive movement and hence does not distinguish between neural and non-neural components of hypertonia. For example, patients early after a stroke may start with increased muscle tone on a neural (spastic) basis, only to develop advanced stiffness and contracture later, resulting in a similar finding of increased resistance that now has a non-neural basis, and this non-neural stiffness may be associated with reduced tonic stretch reflex and tendon jerk activity.

MAS is defined as follows:

0   No increase in muscle tone

1   Slight increase in muscle tone, manifested by a catch and release or by minimal resistance at end range of motion, when the affected part is moved in flexion or extension

1+   Slight increase in muscle tone, manifested by a catch, followed by minimal resistance throughout the remainder (less than half) of range of motion

2   More marked increase in muscle tone through most of the range of motion, but the affected part is easily moved

3   Considerable increase in muscle tone, passive movement is difficult

4   Affected part is rigid in flexion or extension

Tardieu scale

This scale quantifies spasticity by assessing the response of muscle to stretch applied at different velocities. The velocity of stretch ranges from V1 (as slow as possible) to V3 (as fast as possible) and the response of muscle to stretch ranges from 0 (no resistance throughout course of passive movement) to 5 (joint is immobile). The Tardieu scale may be more sensitive in detecting spasticity from contractures compared to the MAS (Patrick and Ada, 2006).

Joint range of motion

Passive and active joint range of motion can be measured.

Measures of function

     a. Pain: numerical pain rating scale

     b. Passive function

     c. Active function

     d. Spasms: frequency of spasms can be measured (e.g. Penn Spasm Frequency Scale)

Other assessment scale

Goal Attainment Scale (GAS)

Patients set their own goals of spasticity treatment in conjunction with the treating healthcare team. Results of intervention are scored from -2 to +2:

0   outcome as expected

+1 to +2   outcome better than expected

-1 to -2   outcome worse than expected

This yields a numeric score that allows for analysing group performance. It is criterion-referenced rather than norm-referenced, making it responsive to minimally clinically significant changes.

Management of spasticity

Is spasticity symptomatic?

Define the problem that is affecting the patient. Is it causing pain or affecting passive and/or active function? Input from the patient's carers and managing healthcare team is useful. Some of the aims of spasticity treatment include:

- Relief of pain and discomfort

- Improvement of posture

- Facilitation of sitting, standing, and walking

- Reduction in burden of care

- Improvement of hygiene in areas such as the palm, axilla and groin

- Improvement in body image and self esteem

- Prevention of complications such as pressure ulcers

Is spasticity beneficial?

Spasticity can confer certain benefits. Knee extensor spasticity allows the patient with weak knee extensors to perform transfers, stand and walk.

Are there aggravating factors?

Spasticity can be aggravated by certain conditions and noxious stimuli and these must be ruled out/treated before further adjustments in spasticity management are considered. These factors are mentioned in Table 2.

Table 2. Aggravating factors for spasticity.

Skin lesions	• Pressure sores
	• Local skin infection or irritation
	• Ingrown toe nails
Urinary tract dysfunction	• Infection
	• Urinary tract stones
	• Incomplete bladder emptying/retention
Gastro-intestinal dysfunction	• Constipation
	• Diarrhoea
	• Overflow incontinence
Central nervous system	• Cerebrovascular disease, further stroke/transient ischemic attack (TIA)
	• Hydrocephalus
	• Syrinx development
Systemic illness	• Generalised infection
	• Deep venous thrombosis
Drugs	• Rapid withdrawal of anti-spasticity drugs
Others	• Stress, pain during menstruation

Treatment of spasticity

Accurate pre-intervention assessment and intensive post-rehabilitation therapy are crucial for successful management of the patients with symptomatic spasticity and this invariably would involve a multidisciplinary team.

Physical therapy

Physical therapy includes:

- Stretching: prolonged, sustained stretching to improve the viscoelastic properties of the muscle-tendon unit and its extensibility

- Casting: a stretching method that immobilises the limb in the stretched position to induce prolonged muscle stretching. Serial casting involves the stepwise application of a plaster or fiberglass cast applied around a joint. The repeated application of casts with the joint being stretched further with each application leads to an improved range of motion, increased function, and/or decreased pain
- Proper positioning and seating
- Muscle strengthening and re-education

Physical modalities

Various physical modalities have been used to reduce spasticity. These include cryotherapy, heat therapy and electrical stimulation. The evidence thus far suggests that functional electrical stimulation and transcutaneous nerve stimulation (TENS) are probably effective in reducing spasticity.

Orthotic splints

Resting upper and lower limb splints are frequently used to reduce or prevent worsening of spasticity. Donning and doffing as well as skin breakdown are issues to be considered before prescribing splints.

Pharmacological treatment

Table 3. Pharmacological treatment of spasticity.

Drug	Dose	Administration	Mechanism of action	Side-effects
Benzo-diazepines e.g. Diazepam	5–20 mg TDS	Oral	Increases the affinity of GABA for the GABA receptor complex leading to an increase in presynaptic inhibition and reduction of synaptic reflexes	Sedation, weakness, hypotension, confusion, depression and ataxia, risk of addiction with prolonged use

Clonazepam	0.5–1.0 mg OD	Oral	Same as diazepam	same as Diazepam
Gabapentin	2400–3600 mg daily	Oral	Structurally similar to GABA; Increases brain level of GABA	Somnolence, nystagmus, ataxia, headache, tremor
Baclofen	5–20 mg TDS-QDS	Oral	Centrally acting GABA analogue; binds to GABA b receptor at the presynaptic terminal and inhibits muscle stretch reflex	Sedation, dizziness, weakness, fatigue, nausea. Lowers seizure threshold
Tizanidine	4–36 mg daily	Oral	Imidazole derivative, with agonist action on alpha-2 adrenergic receptors in central nervous system	Sedation, dizziness, mild hypotension, weakness, hepatotoxicity
Dantrolene	25–100 mg QDS	Oral	Interferes with the release of calcium from sarcoplasmic reticulum of muscles	Generalised muscle weakness, mild sedation, dizziness, nausea, hepatotoxicity

Medications are generally considered for patients with generalised spasticity. Those with centrally acting side effects, especially the benzodiazepines, should be avoided in stroke and brain injury, as they can cause sedation and cognitive impairments.

Chemodenervation treatment

Chemodenervation treatment is the recommended treatment for focal spasticity.

Nerve blocks

The selected nerve is injected with a neurolytic agent, either phenol 5–7% or ethyl alcohol (45–100%), under guidance of a nerve stimulator. Side-effects include pain during injection and dysesthesia due to destruction of sensory nerve fibres. Hence it is most useful in predominantly motor nerves. These include the obturator nerve (adductor spasticity aiding personal hygiene and catheter care) and musculocutaneous nerve (elbow flexor spasticity).

Botulinum toxin injection

Botulinum is a neurotoxin which causes neuromuscular blockade by blocking the pre-synaptic release of acetylcholine resulting in muscle paralysis. The toxin is produced by *Clostridium botulinum* and seven strains of the bacterium have been identified, labelled A–G. Toxin-A (Botox®, Dysport®, and Xeomin®) is the serotype that has been developed into a therapeutic agent and widely applied in clinical practice. Botulinum toxin-B (Neurobloc®) is also available. However, it is less frequently used due to its shorter duration of action. Units and dosing for different brands of botulinum toxin-A are not interchangeable and are therefore specific to the brand.

It is injected intramuscularly and muscles to be injected are identified either via muscle palpation, electromyography, electrical stimulation or ultrasound. Therapeutic effect is seen in 7–10 days, peaks in 4–6 weeks and wanes by 12 weeks. Serious adverse events are uncommon and include local and distant muscle weakness.

Surgical treatment

Intrathecal baclofen pump

Intrathecal baclofen directly acts on GABA receptors in the lumbar spinal cord where a high concentration of receptors allows small doses to be used to good effect without systemic side effects. The intrathecal baclofen pump both stores and delivers programmable doses of baclofen through a catheter into the spinal subarachnoid space. It is indicated for carefully selected patients with significant spasticity who do not respond to other treatment.

Procedure related complications include infection, skin erosions, and cerebrospinal fluid leak and seroma formation around the pump. Abrupt withdrawal of intrathecal baclofen due to pump failure, battery failure, catheter block, or patient non-compliance to treatment can cause a clinical emergency, with features similar to the neuroleptic malignant syndrome which includes high fever, confusion, rebound spasticity, and muscle rigidity.

Orthopaedic intervention

This include tendon release (tenotomy) for patients with severe fixed contractures and tendon transfers. Examples include tendon Achilles release for plantarflexion contractures, and SPLATT (split anterior tibial tendon transfer) procedure for correction of ankle inversion.

References

- Lance JW. The control of muscle tone, reflexes, and movement: Robert Wartenberg lecture. Neurology 1980;30:1303–1313.

- Nathan P. Some comments on spasticity and rigidity. In: New developments in electromyography and clinical neurophysiology, Desmedt JE (Ed). Karger, Basel, Switzerland. 1973;13–14.

- Patrick E, Ada L. The Tardieu Scale differentiates contracture from spasticity whereas the Ashworth Scale is confounded by it. Clin Rehabil 2006;20(2):173–182.

15

Medical Emergencies and Complications in Rehabilitation

RAJESWARAN Deshan Kumar

Chest pain

- Important to always have a good history and tailored physical examination
- Exclude life threatening causes first

Causes

- Acute myocardial infarction (AMI)
  - Pain usually squeezing, burning and radiates to neck/left arm. Associated with shortness of breath
  - Ask for previous symptoms of angina (chest pain with exertion)
  - Look for risk factors (diabetes, hypertension, hyperlipidemia, age, obesity, smoking, family history, drug use, e.g. cocaine)
  - Can have atypical presentation (epigastric pain with nausea, anxiety, syncope, shortness of breath) in elderly and diabetic patients (silent infarcts)

- Aortic dissection
  - Pain is sudden, maximum at onset, tearing/ripping and radiates to back
  - Risk factors of hypertension, history of chest trauma, coarctation of aorta, connective tissue disorders
  - Look for delay (radio-radial or radio-femoral) of pulses or lower systolic blood pressure in one limb

- Pulmonary embolism
  - Look for history of immobilisation (> 3 days), recent surgery, deep vein thrombosis, spinal cord injury, malignancy, hypercoagulable state, contraceptive pill use

- Pneumonia

- Pneumothorax

- Musculoskeletal

  - Recent trauma/fracture of ribs

  - Costochondritis

  - Pain usually worse with palpation or movement

- Gastroesophageal reflux disease (GERD)

  - Burning sensation, bitter taste in mouth, worse on lying down and with certain foods

- Peptic ulcer disease

- Herpes zoster (pain can be prodromal and precede the onset of vesicles)

- Anxiety attack

Initial investigation approach

- The history and physical examination will guide the appropriate investigations to order

- Ensure vital signs are stable (i.e. blood pressure (BP), pulse rate, oxygen saturation (SpO2) via pulse oximetry

- Obtain 12 lead electrocardiogram (ECG)

- ST segment elevation (≥ 1 mm in 2 or more leads) or ST segment depression (≥ 0.5 mm) indicative of acute coronary syndrome (ACS)

- Compare with old ECG to see if changes are new

- Sinus tachycardia, right bundle branch block suggestive of pulmonary embolism. Occasionally can have S1Q3T3 but less specific

- Full blood count, cardiac enzymes (creatinine kinase, creatinine kinase-MB, troponin I)

- Renal panel, prothrombin time/activated partial thromboplastin time (PT/APTT) (baseline)

- D-dimer: if pulmonary embolism is suspected; negative test rules it out; however, it can be elevated with recent surgery, trauma, inflammation, malignancy

- If ECG does not have abnormalities but patient has risk factors for ACS—to continue serial ECG and cardiac examination (6–8 hourly) over the next 12–16 hours

- Chest X-ray (CXR) to look for pneumothorax, pneumonia, widened mediastinum suggestive of dissection

- CT pulmonary angiogram (CTPA): to exclude pulmonary embolism (especially if d-dimer raised). To consider monitoring and stabilization in acute setting till therapeutic anticoagulation is achieved

- CT aortogram: to exclude aortic dissection

Management

- If suspect ACS, give O2, S/L 0.6 mg GTN (glyceryl trinitrate) and analgesia to relief pain

- Aspirin 300 mg stat

- Beta blocker

- To consult cardiologist if any suspicion or evidence of angina/AMI based on history, physical examination, ECG and laboratory tests for further investigations, treatment and monitoring

- If pulmonary embolism, ensure supplemental oxygen, IV fluid resuscitation and start anticoagulation (subcutaneous low molecular weight heparinoids, e.g. Clexane) if no contraindication

- Need closer monitoring in acute setting (especially large pulmonary embolism) till therapeutic anticoagulation is reached

- If suspect aortic dissection, ensure hemodynamic stability 1before confirming with appropriate investigations

Hypertension

- BP > 140/90 mmHg

- Need to check if patient is a known hypertensive and if is on usual hypertensive medications

- Look for any source of pain which can contribute to the hypertension

- Need to check if patient recently had a stroke. Loss of cerebral autoregulation can result in high BP early post stroke

- For hemorrhagic stroke, can aim to control BP to < 140/90 mmHg
- For ischemic stroke (especially if patient has significant carotid artery stenosis) need to be cautious about lowering BP too aggressively in first 2 weeks post stroke
- Need to balance the benefit between immediate decrease in BP against the risk of significant decrease in cerebral perfusion which can lead to progression of the stroke/new infarcts
- For ischemic stroke can aim to control BP to about 180 mmHg systolic within the first 2 weeks before tightening control
- Need to look for signs of end organ damage (heart failure, AMI, renal impairment, papilloedema, hypertensive encephalopathy) to guide management and choice of antihypertensives
- To consider looking for secondary causes of hypertension especially in young patients (e.g. pheochromocytoma, Conn's syndrome, thyroid dysfunction, coarctation of aorta, Cushing's syndrome, acromegaly)

Autonomic dysreflexia (AD)

- Refer to chapter 4, Spinal Cord Injury Rehabilitation

Hypotension

- Look for features of shock (tachycardia, dyspnea, cool peripheries, chest pain, oliguria)
- Causes
    - Bleeding gastrointestinal tract
    - Severe dehydration
    - Cardiac failure
    - Arrhythmia
    - Sepsis
    - Spinal shock
    - Medications (anti-hypertensives)

Initial investigation approach

- Full blood count, renal panel, liver function test, cardiac enzymes, disseminated intravascular coagulopathy screen

- Arterial blood gas (ABG), lactate (if needed)

- Group and cross match (GXM)

- Urine FEME (full and microscopic examination), c/s (culture and sensitivity)

- Blood culture and sensitivity

- 12 lead ECG

- CXR (depending on symptoms)

Management

- Shock needs to be treated immediately. Check ABC

- Supplemental oxygen

- 2 large bore IV lines

- Run intravenous fluids (normal saline/Hartmann's)

- Watch for BP response after fluid resuscitation to guide management

- Consider inotropes if BP not responsive to adequate fluid resuscitation

- IV antibiotics to treat source of sepsis

- IV packed cell transfusion if any indication of bleeding gastrointestinal tract/ anemia (Hb < 7 g/dL)

- To consider CTPA (if suspicion of pulmonary embolism)

- Will need monitoring in acute setting

- To consider appropriate referral (e.g. to cardiologist if cause is arrhythmias, AMI, heart failure)

Shortness of breath

Main differential diagnoses

- Pulmonary embolism

- AMI

- Congestive heart failure/acute pulmonary edema

- Asthma/chronic obstructive airways disease exacerbation

- Anemia

- Pre shock/shock

- Targeted history and physical exam. Look for history of ischemic heart disease (with poor ejection fraction), congestive heart failure, airways disease (e.g. asthma, chronic obstructive airways disease)

- If patient is dysphagic/with nasogastric tube: consider possibility of aspiration pneumonia

- Any associated chest pain

- Check pulse rate for any tachyarrhythmia (e.g. atrial fibrillation) leading to heart failure

- Examine if patient is able to speak full sentences, any accessory muscles of respiration used/deviated trachea/crepitations/rhonchi/reduced air entry

Initial investigation approach

- Full blood count, renal panel, cardiac enzymes

- D-dimer (if suspicion of pulmonary embolism)

- ECG

- CXR

Management

- Assess ABC

- Check SpO2. Give supplemental oxygen if needed

- If suspect PE/AMI—refer to previous section on "chest pain" for management

- If in fluid overload—intravenous Frusemide to diurese and monitor intake/output strictly

- If asthma/chronic obstructive airways disease—to institute nebulized bronchodilators accordingly and steroids (intravenous hydrocortisone/oral prednisolone)

Bleeding gastrointestinal tract (BGIT)

- Ensure patient is clinically stable

- Significant risk factors (age, anticoagulation, antiplatelets, non-steroidal anti-inflammatory drug (NSAID) use, stress from injury/recent illness, history of diverticulosis, hemorrhoids, liver disease/cirrhosis, alcohol abuse and peptic ulcer disease)

- Upper GIT causes: peptic ulcer disease, gastritis, Cushing's ulcers, esophagitis, esophageal ulcers, varices, aortoenteral fistula

- Lower GIT causes: diverticular disease, hemorrhoids, rectal ulcer

- Physical exam to look for signs of hypotension, tachycardia, liver disease (jaundice, spider nevi, palmar erythema, hepatosplenomegaly)

- Per rectal exam—look for fresh bleeding, melena, hemorrhoids

Initial investigation approach

- Full blood count, renal panel, liver function test, PT/PTT, GXM

Management

- Ensure large bore intravenous plugs for fluid resuscitation

- Nil by mouth. Stop anticoagulants/antiplatelets

- Intravenous normal saline/Hartmann's solution initially

- Intravenous Nexium (esomeprazole) 40 mg stat and then followed by Nexium infusion (8 mg/h)

- Correct coagulopathy with fresh frozen plasma (FFP)

- Packed cell transfusion

- To consult gastroenterologist for further investigation (gastroscopy/colonoscopy) and monitoring of condition in acute setting

Altered mental status

- Check ABC (ensure patient can protect airway and not in respiratory distress) and ensure vital signs are stable (hypotension can cause cerebral hypoperfusion)
- General examination to look for signs of sepsis
- Check if any history of seizures witnessed
- Neurological examination to look for focal neurological signs (e.g. lateralized weakness, pupillary reflexes, eye movements/ version, plantar responses)

Differential diagnoses

- Central nervous system event – stroke, post seizure/ non-convulsive status epilepticus
- Endocrine — hypoglycemia , hypo/hyperthyroidism, adrenal insufficiency
- Infection — sepsis
- Electrolyte abnormalities — hypo/hypernatremia, hypo/hypercalcemia
- Respiratory — hypercapnia (type II respiratory failure), hypoxia
- Drugs (benzodiazepines, antihistamines, tricyclic antidepressants, antipsychotics, baclofen, gabapentin, anticonvulsants)
- Urine retention/constipation (especially in elderly)

Initial investigation approach

- Full blood count, renal panel, calcium, liver function test, thyroid function test
- Stat hypocount
- ABG
- Drug levels of anticonvulsants (e.g. phenytoin toxicity)
- Urine analysis (UFEME) and culture and sensitivity (c/s), blood culture and sensitivity (c/s) (if febrile)
- ECG and cardiac enzymes (atypical presentation of AMI)

- CXR — to exclude pneumonia (especially in elderly)
- CT/MRI brain — if there are new neurological deficits to exclude new stroke/worsening hydrocephalus
- Electroencephalogram (EEG) — if considering non-convulsive status epilepticus

Management

- Ensure ABC
- Supplemental oxygen if hypoxic/ BIPAP (bilevel positive airway pressure; with monitoring in acute setting) if type II respiratory failure and CO_2 retention
- Intravenous fluids if hypotensive
- Cover with intravenous antibiotics if suspect sepsis as cause
- Clear bowels and ensure no urine retention
- Titrate or stop any medications that can contribute to altered mental status

Seizures

- Has patient ever had seizures before? Is patient on anticonvulsants?
- Any history of alcohol withdrawal, sedative/benzodiazepine use?
- History of diabetes mellitus (DM)/on oral hypoglycemic agents
- Was seizure focal or generalized?
- Any history of stroke/traumatic brain injury (common complication)?

Investigation approach

- Full blood count, renal panel, liver function test
- Drug levels of anticonvulsants (e.g. phenytoin) if patient taking it
- CT brain—to look for any new intracranial event (e.g. hemorrhage/infarct)

Management

- To support airway, breathing, circulation and prevent self inflicted injury

- Follow through workup to determine the cause and institute appropriate management

- Ensure patient is lying in left lateral position with suction device ready to prevent aspiration

- Do not interfere if patient is spontaneously breathing or force anything into the mouth

- Establish IV access as soon as possible

- Check hypocount and correct with intravenous dextrose 50% 40 ml if hypoglycemic

- Most seizures abort within 3 min. If second seizure or status epilepticus then give intravenous diazepam 10 mg stat / rectal diazepam 10 mg (if no intravenous access available) stat

- Then load intravenous phenytoin (20 mg/kg) with ECG and close BP monitoring

- To monitor in acute setting for patients with status epilepticus

Electrolyte abnormalities

Hyponatremia

- Serum Na+ < 135 mmol/L (usually no symptoms till less than 125 mmol/L)

- Is the patient symptomatic—lethargy, muscle cramps, altered mental status, nausea/vomiting, seizures, altered consciousness

- What were the recent sodium levels? (To determine acuity of change)

- Is there any evidence of volume depletion? (Orthostatic hypotension with appropriate response tachycardia)

- Any history of vomiting or diarrhea?

- Any history of cardiac, renal or liver failure?

Investigation approach

- Exclude pseudohyponatremia (due to hyperglycemia, hyperproteinemia, severe hyperlipidemia) or laboratory error (especially if very low values and patient is asymptomatic)

- Assess patient's volume status (skin turgor, mucosa, jugular venous pressure, fluid balance on input-output charts)

- Check serum sodium, serum osmolality, urine sodium (spot), urine osmolality (spot)

- Other laboaratory investigations if clinically indicated (thyroid function test, 8 am cortisol, liver panel, renal panel)

Euvolemic

- Syndrome of inappropriate anti diuretic hormone (SIADH) where urine osmolality inappropriately high (> 300 mOsm/kg) for serum osmolality (< 290 mOsm/kg) and urine Na+ usually > 20 mmol/L.

- Causes of SIADH include stroke, head injury, pneumonia and drugs (e.g. selective serotonin reuptake inhibitors, e.g fluoxetine, tricyclic antidepressants, and antipsychotics)

- Hypothyroidism

- Glucocorticoid deficiency

Hypovolemic

- Urine Na+ < 10 mmol/L [in gastrointestinal (vomiting and diarrhea) and third space losses] and > 20 mmol/L (in renal losses due to diuretics like thiazides, adrenal insufficiency, salt losing nephritis, severe hyperglycemia)

Hypervolemic

- Due to cardiac failure, renal failure, liver cirrhosis

Management

- Treat the underlying cause

- Intravenous crystalloids (e.g. 0.9% normal saline) for hypovolemic patients till volume replete

- Free water restriction (800–1000 ml/day) for hypervolemic and euvolemic patients

- Salt loading with salt tablets can be considered (NaCl tab 2 tds) in hypovolemic and euvolemic patients

- Consider the use of loop diuretics (frusemide) especially in hypervolemic states or for patients with SIADH who do not respond to free water restriction and sodium tablets

- If patient is symptomatic (e.g. seizures or drop in level of consciousness), correct with IV 3% normal saline. Aim to correct not more than 8–10 mmol/day to avoid central pontine myelenolysis or pulmonary edema. This should be done in the acute setting with close monitoring of sodium level and neurological status

Hypernatremia

- Serum sodium > 145 mmol/L. Severe symptoms usually do not occur with values < 155 mmol/L

- Check for gastrointestinal (GI) losses (from diarrhea and vomiting), renal losses (diabetes insipidus, administration of diuretics, osmotic diuresis from severe hyperglycemia or mannitol), cutaneous losses (fever, sweating)

- Administration of exogenous steroids or salt tablets?

- Is patient dehydrated? (Inadequate access to water as bedbound, inadequate thirst mechanism)

- Is patient symptomatic? (Lethargy, weakness, seizures, drop in level of consciousness)

- Is patient hypovolemic (loss of hypotonic fluids), euvolemic (net loss of free water) or hypervolemic (gain of hypertonic fluids)?

Investigation approach

- Serum sodium

- Serum osmolality

- Urine sodium (spot)

- Urine osmolality (spot)

Management

- Restore intravascular volume in hypovolemic patients with isotonic intravenous fluids

- Replace free water deficit once euvolemia reached with water or intravenous D5W (5% dextrose in water)/IV 0.45% normal saline if patient unable to take orally

- Do not correct more than 8–10 mmol/L in a day to avoid cerebral edema

- Treat underlying conditions (e.g. diabetes insipidus)

Hypokalemia

- Serum potassium < 3.5 mmol/L
- Usually due to GI losses (diarrhea, vomiting) or side effects from medications (diuretics, beta-2 agonists)
- Usually symptomatic when < 3.0 mmol/L
- Look for symptoms such as muscle weakness (can involve respiratory muscles), ileus, nausea, vomiting, abdomen distension, rhabdomyolysis

Investigation approach

- Serum potassium
- Serum magnesium (hypomagnesemia can occur in up to 40% of cases and must be replaced concurrently with potassium)
- Spot urine potassium
- 12 lead ECG (when serum K+ < 2.5 mmol/L)

Management

- Need to correct rapidly (especially when K+ < 2.5 mmol/L) to prevent malignant cardiac arrhythmias. Also important in patients with preexisting cardiac disease or on medications like digoxin
- If serum K+ is between 2.5–3.4 mmol/L, can replace orally if no significant heart disease or concurrent digoxin treatment. Can give span K 1.2 g tds or mixture KCl 10–20 mls tds. If unable to take orally, then correct intravenously
- If symptomatic or serum K+ < 2.5 mmol/L, correct intravenously (intravenous 10 mmol KCl in 100 ml 0.9% normal saline over 1 hour. Repeat this cycle once or twice before checking serum K+)

Hyperkalemia

- Serum potassium > 5.0 mmol/L

Causes

- Acute/chronic kidney disease

- Adverse effects of medications [e.g. ACE (angiotensin converting enzyme) inhibitors, angiotensin receptor blockers, potassium sparing diuretics]

- Strenuous exercise, rhabdomyolysis

- Trauma

- Symptoms with severe hyperkalemia include muscle weakness and paralysis, cardiac arrhythmias

Investigation approach

- Need to exclude pseudohyperkalemia during blood collection (e.g. difficult venipuncture, excessive vacuum force, tight tourniquet, delay in processing time of specimen)

- 12 lead ECG (when serum K+ > 5.5mmol/L). Look for peaked T waves, prolonged PR interval, flattened P waves and widened QRS complex. This can evolve to ventricular tachycardia, ventricular fibrillation and asystole

- Check baseline hypocount

Management

- If serum K+ > 6.5 mmol/L, any ECG changes or high risk patients (acute renal failure, end stage renal failure on dialysis, coronary artery disease, acute myocardial injury), then give 10 ml of intravenous calcium gluconate 10% over 2–3 min (to stabilize the cardiac membrane). Can give slow infusion over 20 min in 100 ml of dextrose 5% in patients on digoxin

- Intravenous dextrose 50% 40 ml (to prevent hypoglycemia) + intravenous regular insulin 5–10 units (for transcellular shift of K+). If baseline hypocount > 18 mmol/L, can omit the intravenous dextrose 50% bolus. If baseline hypocount < 6 mmol/L or NBM/poor oral intake/previous episodes of hypoglycemia, then consider a maintenance intravenous dextrose infusion

- Enhance clearance of potassium from the body through ion exchange resin (Resonium PO 15–30 g q8h or enema 30 g q 8h)

- Can consider beta agonist nebulizer, e.g. salbutamol or intravenous Frusemide (for patients with residual renal function)

- Check hypocount hourly for 6 hours after this and serum potassium 2 hours later to document efficacy

- Need to repeat ECG 10 min after intravenous calcium gluconate given to document resolution of changes and another one in 30–60 min. Can consider another dose of intravenous calcium gluconate if ECG changes still persistent

- If these measures are ineffective (especially in acute kidney injury or renal failure) then consider referral to nephrologist for haemodialysis

Hypoglycemia

- Hypocount < 4.0 mmol/L (DM patient)
- Adrenergic symptoms—palpitations, tremor, diaphoresis
- Beta blockers can mask the adrenergic symptoms (hypertension, tachycardia) except diaphoresis
- Neuroglycopenic symptoms—reduced mentation, confusion, focal neurological deficit, seizures, coma
- Patients with long standing DM may lose ability to perceive hypoglycemia
- Potential complication in patients with DM (on oral hypoglycemics/insulin) with poor oral intake and also due to increasing energy requirements with exercise
- Impaired renal function can affect clearance of insulin

Management

- If hypocount between 3–4 mmol/L and patient asymptomatic, then adjust DM medications
- If hypocount < 3 mmol/L or patient symptomatic (adrenergic symptoms) and conscious—can give oral glucose drink quickly and monitor hypocount in 30 min
- If any neuroglycopenic symptoms, give intravenous dextrose 50% 40 ml and then followed by intravenous dextrose 10% 500 ml over 8 hours
- Monitor hypocount hourly till stable
- Keep intravenous dextrose maintenance till patient able to eat well orally

Hyperglycemia

- Need to ensure patient is stable and no signs of diabetic ketoacidosis/ hyperosmolar hyperglycemic state(HHS)

- HHS usually in DM patient with concomitant illness and poor oral intake

- Usually due to inadequate insulin/oral hypoglycemic dose—need to titrate accordingly to manage high glucose levels

- Can also be due to stress from infection, oral glucocorticoids (e.g. prednisolone) or poor dietary compliance in patients

Fever

- Temperature > 38°C

- Consider the following differential diagnosis and tailor history and physical examination to look for the following:

Infectious causes

- Urinary tract infections (especially catheter associated)
    - Presents with dysuria, frequency, suprapubic or pelvic discomfort, hematuria, renal angle tenderness (need to exclude pyelonephritis)
    - Can also present with increase in spasticity or autonomic dysreflexia (in spinal cord injured patients)

- Pneumonia
    - Increased cough, purulent sputum, hypoxia
    - Common in patients with stroke/brain injury with dysphagia (prone to aspiration of saliva) as well as in high tetraplegics and recumbent patients

- Skin and soft tissue infections
    - Look for breaks in the skin/web spaces (especially in diabetics or immunocompromised patients) for signs of cellulitis
    - Examine any amputee stump wounds/surgical incision sites to look for poor healing, erythema, tenderness, purulent discharge
    - Look for secondarily infected pressure ulcers (erythematous, sloughy base with purulent discharge, poor healing)
    - Grade 4 pressure ulcers can involve the bone and result in osteomyelitis
    - Check any intravenous plug sites for thrombophlebitis

- Sinusitis

- High index of suspicion in patients with nasogastric tubes
- Intraabdominal/pelvic source of infection
    - Peritoneal signs may be attenuated in spinal cord injury patients with high thoracic/cervical injuries. Therefore, may need to look for other signs (e.g. autonomic dysreflexia) or consider imaging abdomen if no obvious source from initial workup
    - Hepatobiliary sepsis
    - Abscesses (melioidosis especially in diabetics)
    - Appendicitis
- Endocarditis (check for heart murmurs/signs of heart failure/septic emboli)
- Viral illness
    - Patient can be having a upper respiratory tract infection, influenza or gastroenteritis
- Clostridium difficile colitis
    - Patient would have diarrhea and abdomen cramps
    - Check for recent history of antibiotic use

Non-infectious causes

- Inflammatory conditions (gout, osteoarthritis flare, calcium pyrophosphate deposition disease of joints, rheumatoid arthritis flare)
- Drug fever
- Thromboembolic disease (e.g. deep vein thrombosis, pulmonary embolism)
- Paroxysmal autonomic instability (especially in severe brain injury and can be associated with dystonia)
- Can occasionally be associated with autonomic dysreflexia in SCI
- Heterotopic ossification
- Malignancy

Initial investigation workup

- Full blood count, C-reactive protein (CRP), procalcitonin
- Liver function test

- Renal function

- UFEME , urine c/s (obtain from freshly placed catheter or mid-stream urine sample)

- Blood c/s × 2 sets

- Stool for leucocyte, c/s, Clostridium difficile toxin (if presenting with diarrhea/ bloody stools)

- CXR

- Joint aspirate (if joint swelling present and to exclude septic arthritis/confirm etiology)

- Wound c/s (if purulent discharge present)

- Deep tissue culture/biopsy (for osteomyelitis/infected pressure ulcers)

- Imaging studies (e.g. ultrasound/CT abdomen or Doppler lower limb) may be required if source of infection not clearly identified from initial workup

Management

- Ensure vital signs stable and no signs of septic shock

- Look for any potential indwelling intravenous plug or catheter that can be the source of infection and ensure it has been changed

- Anti-pyretics (e.g. paracetamol)

- Can consider NSAIDS (e.g. voltaren) for inflammatory conditions, autonomic dysfunction and for analgesia (in cases of gout/osteoarthritis flare)

- Consider colchicine if suspect gout flare

- Ensure adequate fluid resuscitation

- Start empiric antibiotics (ensure septic workup done prior to this) based on clinical suspicion of likely source of infection (to follow institution based antibiotic guidelines for selection of empiric antibiotics)

16

Walking Aids and Lower Limb Orthotics

LIM Pang Hung

Walking aids

Reasons for use

1. For support: when independent lower limb support of body weight is ineffective due to

   - Significant strength reduction

   - Pain limiting movement and weight bearing

   - Lower limb fracture

2. For balance assistance: when postural control is inadequate and/or balance reaction speed is reduced due to

   - Aging

   - Deconditioning from prolonged bed rest, inactivity

   - Sensory deficits in vision, vestibular or somatosensory systems

   - Movement disorders such as ataxia or apraxia

Types of walking aids

1. **Axillary crutches (height adjustable)**

   - Purpose

     - Most commonly used for to assist body weight support

     - Not suitable for patients with poor balance

   - Indications

     - Lower limb fractures or joint surgery, requiring partial weight bearing or non-weight bearing of affected leg

- Lower limb amputation (for pre-prosthetic fitting ambulation or early stage prosthetic leg gait training)
- Musculoskeletal injuries to lower limb (e.g. ankle or knee sprain)
  - Advantage
    - Easier to use (than elbow crutches)
    - Preferred by patients with weak upper limb extensor strength

2. **Elbow crutches**
  - Purpose
    - As per axillary crutches
    - Not suitable for patients who have weak upper limb extensor strength
  - Indications
    - As per axillary crutches
  - Advantage
    - Lighter than axillary crutches
    - Easier to manoeuvre at steps and kerbs
    - More trendy designs and colours to choose from

3. **Forearm gutter crutch (see Fig. 1)**
  - Purpose
    - To be swapped with one side of the axillary or elbow crutches
    - Not suitable for patients with poor balance
  - Indications
    - As per axillary crutches
    - When patient is unable to bear weight through his or her wrist and hand due to injury
  - Advantage
    - Avoidance of weight through injured wrist and hand while still using proximal shoulder extensor muscles for assistance in weight bearing

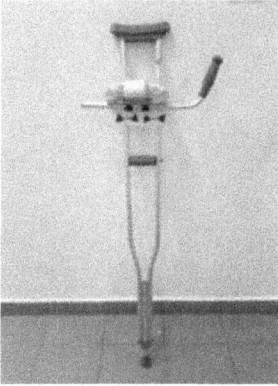

Fig. 1. Forearm gutter crutch.

4. **Walking Frames (height adjustable)**

(i) Regular

- Purpose
  - Commonly used by persons who require help in "body weight support" and/or for stabilising postural control
- Indications
  - Lower limb fractures or joint surgery, requiring partial weight bearing or non-weight bearing of affected leg
  - Lower limb amputation (for pre-prosthetic fitting ambulation or early stage prosthetic leg gait training)
  - Musculoskeletal injuries to lower limb (e.g. ankle or knee sprain)
  - Patients with neurological conditions causing lower limb weakness and/or poor balance
  - Frail and weak patients
- Advantage
  - Enhance postural stability due to an expanded base of support over four points

(ii) Rollator walking frame variant (2 wheeled)

- Purpose
  - As per standard walking frame (regular)

- Set of front wheels allow pushing and gliding of the walking frame over ground hence avoiding actions of lifting and placing of the frame
- Indications
  - As per standard walking frame (regular)
- Advantage
  - For persons who are very weak and/or are unable to lift up the walking frame during walking
  - For persons who have poor balance requiring the expanded base of support at all times when walking

5. **Walking stick**

   (i) Regular (height adjustable)
   - Purpose
     - Modestly stabilising patient's postural control
     - Small amount of body weight support is possible
   - Indications
     - Mild musculoskeletal injuries to lower limb (e.g. ankle or knee sprain)
     - Mild stroke causing unilateral bodily weakness
     - Need for increased patient's confidence and safety when walking in challenging multi-tasking outdoor environment
   - Advantage
     - A light walking aid, easy to carry about

   (ii) Umbrella (with rubber tip, fixed height)
   - Purpose
     - As per walking stick (regular)
   - Indications
     - As per walking stick (regular)
   - Advantages
     - Less stigmatising look

   (iii) Hiking pole (height adjustable)

- Purpose
  - As per walking stick (regular)
- Indications
  - As per walking stick (regular)
- Advantage
  - Holding onto the vertically oriented handle bar (instead of the usual horizontal handle bar) leads to a more symmetrical postural alignment

6. **Quad stick (height adjustable)**

- Purpose
  - Useful for both "body weight support" and postural stability assistance, especially in neurological hemiplegic conditions
- Indications
  - Persons with hemiplegic neurological weakness and poor balance
  - Lower limb amputation (gait training with prosthetic leg)
  - Musculoskeletal injuries to lower limb (e.g. ankle or knee sprain)
  - When walking stick is inadequate at stabilising or supporting patient
- Advantage
  - Good stability aid resulting from an expanded unilateral base of support
  - Allows compensation of strength and balance to be derived from the less affected side of the body

7. **Platform/forearm support rollator walking frames (height adjustable/ four wheeled)**

- Purpose
  - To assist in heavy leaning body weight support during ambulation training
  - To assist with postural stabilization during ambulation training
- Indications
  - Patients with pronounced weakness and/or poor balance

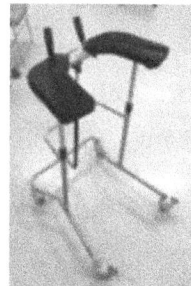

Fig. 2. Platform rollator.

        ◆ Usually used during early stage rehabilitation

    ■ Advantage

        ◆ Enhanced stability resulting from an expanded base of support

        ◆ Substantial body weight support through both upper limbs at elbows

        ◆ Reduces effort of walking over level ground, thereby allowing longer duration of practice

8. Walkers (rollators)

    ■ Purpose

        ◆ A multipurpose walking aid to enhance postural stability and confidence during ambulation

    ■ Indications

        ◆ Older patients with reduced endurance and increased fall risk due to poor balance reaction speed

    ■ Advantage

        ◆ Enhanced stability resulting from an expanded base of support

        ◆ Castor wheels allow for minimal effort in pushing walker (rollator)

        ◆ Resting seat is incorporated in walker design

        ◆ Designed for in- and outdoor use

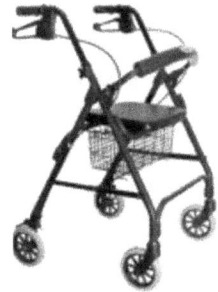

Fig. 3. Walker.

Rule of thumb for setting walking aid height

- Walking aid handle height should usually be at the patient's wrist level in the standing position

Coordinated gait pattern when using crutches

- Walking aids that comes in a pair (e.g. axillary/elbow crutches, holding 2 quad sticks) will have specific coordinated gait patterns to comply with (e.g. 2-point gait pattern, 3-point gait pattern and 4-point gait pattern)

- Coordinated and consistent gait pattern will ensure that the appropriate amount of weight bearing for the affected leg is complied with. Patients are also less likely to trip over themselves due to wrong footing

Stair climbing with walking aid

- General rule of thumb for stair climb is to go up the stairs with the "better leg first" and to get down the stairs with the "weaker leg first"

- Walking aid will usually stay with/or follow the weaker leg during the manoeuvre

Lower limb orthotics

Purpose

- To provide external mechanical support to achieve improved joint alignment so that gait cycle is facilitated

- Names of lower limb orthotics are derived from the joints that the device is applied onto.

Ankle foot orthosis (AFO) variants

1. Posterior leaf splint (spring) AFO (see fig. 4)
   - Usually off the shelf
   - Can also be custom fabricated

2. Supralite AFO (variant of posterior leaf splint)
   - Off the shelf
   - Lightweight and highly flexible

3. Solid AFO (see fig. 5)
   - Custom fabricated

4. Hinged AFO
   - Custom fabricated from a solid AFO

5. Anterior support (Toe-Off) AFO
   - Off the shelf with minor customization possibility
   - Light and strong fibreglass material

6. Ground reaction force AFO
   - Custom fabricated

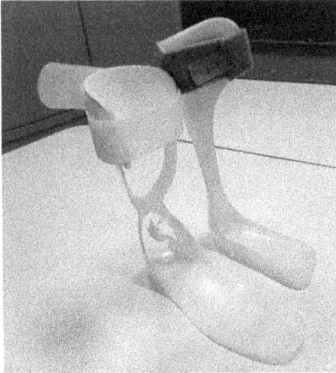

Fig. 4. Posterior leaf splint AFO.

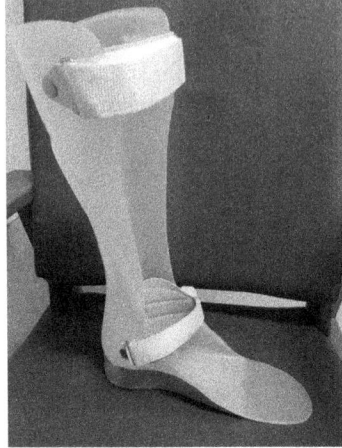

Fig. 5. Solid AFO

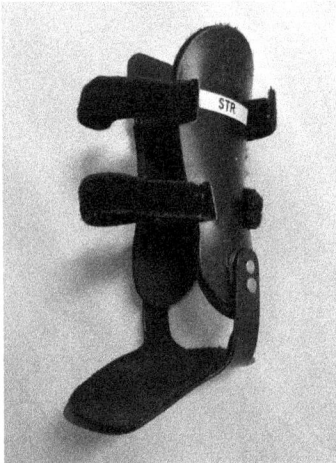

Fig. 6. Surestep.

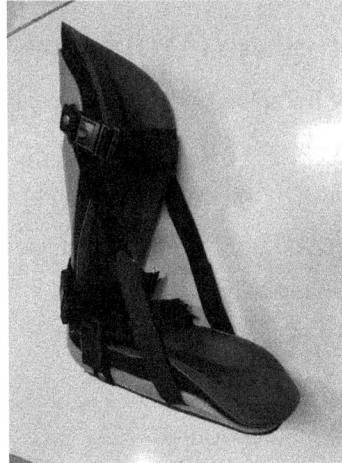

Fig. 7. Resting AFO.

- Specialised custom made AFO to assist patients who are weak at the hip/knee extensors resulting in excessive knee flexion in standing and walking posture (usually the problem occurs bilaterally in both limbs)

7. Surestep, lateral support AFO

- Off the shelf (see Fig. 6)

8. Resting AFO/night splint

- Usually off the shelf but will need custom fabrication if strong spasticity or severe contracture is present (see Fig. 7)

Key considerations in addressing AFO requirements

1. Complexity of joint misalignment encountered during walking

- For simple foot drop correction, foot lifting forces provided through an AFO like the posterior leaf splint, may achieve sufficient ground clearance required during "initial swing" phase in gait

- Complex issues faced during pre-swing in gait cycle may include strong involuntary ankle foot dynamic synergy. This results in twisting action at the forefoot and ankle producing forefoot supination and ankle plantarflexion (equinus foot)

- Such situation may require custom made solid AFO that wraps around the forefoot and ankle to restrict supination and a strong dorsum strap to restrict plantar flexion

- In certain cases, a more flexible off the shelf lateral support AFO like the Sure Step (fixed) AFO may be sufficient to restrict the equinus tendency

2. Step pattern

- Normal gait efficiency is highly derived from the "rear-foot" and "forefoot" rocker mechanisms. In a gait cycle, these mechanisms occur during
  - ◆ Initial contact (initial stance or "heel strike")
  - ◆ Terminal stance ("push-off" or pre-swing)

- All AFOs can allow the rear foot rocker mechanism to take place if the patient has sufficient control and power to generate the forward propulsion momentum, but only AFOs with sufficiently soft and flexible under sole material can allow the forefoot rocker mechanism experience (e.g. the Supralite posterior leaf AFO, or a posterior leaf AFO that has the length of its plastic sole ending just before the ball of the foot)

- The forefoot rocker mechanism is especially important for patients who are progressing in their gait ability, taking larger step lengths and generating higher forward movement momentum

- Specially designed anterior support AFOs are supposed to enhance patient's effort to engage the forefoot rocker mechanism (e.g. the Toe-Off AFO). Such AFOs do require patients to have a sufficient level of strength and control in their gait in order to generate and benefit from the "energy return" offered by the orthotic device during the push off/terminal stance phase in gait

- A solid AFO on the other hand will totally prevent the occurrence of forefoot rocker action

- An alternative method to mimic the forefoot rocker action in the solid AFO is to design and incorporate a hinge that allows dorsiflexion > 90 degrees and stops plantar flexion at about 90 degrees

3. **Ease of wearing**
   - Shape and size of the AFO's sole portion should be slim enough to slip into shoes easily

4. **Comfort**
   - The plastic edges of an AFO must not bend into the skin of the foot and calf
   - Padding should cushion the patient's skin against the AFO material (especially at the weight bearing areas). Otherwise socks should be worn before wearing the AFO

5. **Aesthetics**
   - AFOs should not look excessively bulky and cumbersome

Knee ankle foot orthosis (KAFO)

- Usually prescribed to improve stability of the knee joint as a result of joint laxity or weakness

Knee gaiter

- Usually prescribed to immobilize the affected knee joint during standing or walking tasks
- May also be used for stretching and maintaining knee extension while resting in bed

17
Upper Limb Assistive Devices and Wheelchair Prescription

TOH Ee Mui Shirlene

Introduction

"An Assistive Device is any device that helps someone do something that they might not otherwise be able to do well or at all. Generally, the term is used for devices that help people overcome a handicap such as a mobility, vision, mental, dexterity or hearing loss."

(From: www.nchearingloss.org/assistiv.html)

In general, an assistive device serves the following purposes:

- Increases independence

- Helps to prevent injury

- Protects skin integrity

- Provides support for correct body posture

- Increases level of comfort when performing activities of daily living (ADLs)

The same equipment can be used differently by individuals, depending on their preferences. Some may like the equipment while others may not accept it. When deciding on suitable equipment for prescription and purchase, it is important to discuss this with the occupational and physical therapists, so that the appropriate equipment is prescribed.

This chapter provides an overview of common equipment that individuals with disability may use, in the following order:

- Equipment for ADLs
- Equipment for upper limb positioning and support
- Wheelchairs

Equipment for activities of daily living (ADLs)

Feeding

a. Good grip utensils: soft flexible enlarged handles provide more control for individuals with limited hand control and poor grip

b. Weighted utensils: designed to decrease hand tremors, and allow cutlery to reach the user's mouth easier. Suitable for individual with Parkinson's disease and ataxia

c. Universal cuff: ideal for individuals with good wrist control but has limited or no hand function. Other than slotting a spoon into the universal cuff, other items can be fitted in to perform other activities (a toothbrush or comb)

d. Extensor cuff: used by individuals with poor/no active wrist extension. It aids to stabilise the wrist to provide better distal control and has a small "pocket" to hold small objects such as spoon/fork

Dressing and grooming

a. Button hooks with zipper pull: two aids in one, the hook assists with buttoning needs, and the zipper pull attaches to hard-to-handle zipper tabs, making it easier to zip. Ideal for individuals with poor or no dexterity

b. Long handle reacher: helps to pick up items from the floor and cupboards. Helps with dressing and reaching and grabbing distant objects. Ideal for the elderly, wheelchair users or anyone with walking difficulties, after knee replacement or hip replacement surgery

c. Long handled bath sponge: gives a thorough cleansing of areas where one cannot reach. Suitable for individuals with shoulder and elbow limitations

Meal preparation

a. Angled cooking utensil set: angled handle makes cutting a more natural motion for the wrist. Takes the strain off the wrist and arm while preparing food

b. Swedish cutting board: this tool slices, chops, grates and tenderizes with attached stainless-steel spikes that holds food in place, and a vice is available to secure larger items such as mixing bowls. Suitable for individuals with mobility or dexterity issues and with only one hand use

c. One touch can opener: useful for individuals with bilateral hand weakness

Typing and writing

a. Typing aids: makes typing easier for individuals with significant hand problems. Easily fits on the outside of the hand and allows a full view of the keyboard (see Fig. 1)

b. Page turner: allows individuals with hand weakness to turn book pages themselves by pushing the device against the page

c. Quad writing splint: wraps round the palm and holds the index finger to give individuals with hand weakness, control needed for writing. Designed to hold pencil and pen

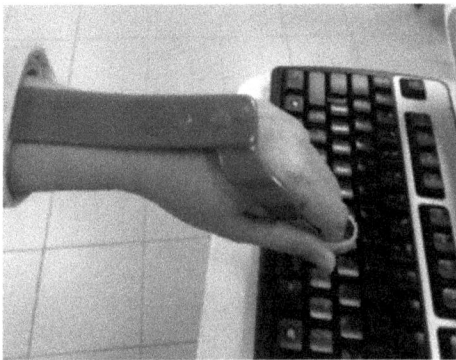

Fig. 1. Typing aid.

Equipment for upper limb positioning and support

a. Forearm resting splint: with wrist commonly positioned in slight extension, metacarpophalangeal and interphalangeal joints in slight flexion, and thumb in opposition (see Fig. 2). It is used to support normal anatomical hand arches, offering resting comfort. Usually used to prevent hand deformities resulting from structural changes associated with neurological conditions, burns, arthritic disease and orthopaedic injuries

b. Anti-spasticity hand splint: wrist is positioned in neutral or slight extension, metacarpophalangeal and interphalangeal joints in slight flexion, and thumb in abduction with 1/3 circumduction. Hand is positioned in this splint to inhibit muscle tone by decreasing the stretch reflex. Splint is fabricated to support hand with moderate spasticity

c. Wrist cock-up splint/wrist brace: wrist is positioned in slight extension. This splint immobilises the wrist and allow fingers manipulation. Immobilisation (for a set period) is for used for reducing acute inflammation of the wrist joint, wrist sprain, and tendonitis and carpal tunnel syndrome

d. Tenodesis splint or thumb spica splint: thumb is positioned in 2/3 cirumduction so as to allow opposition of thumb with index finger. Commonly used to provide support for thumb injuries (ligament instability, sprain or muscle strain), arthritis and thumb sprains. Also used to stabilise the metacarpophalangeal joints in tenodesis training for individuals with spinal cord injury at C6 level

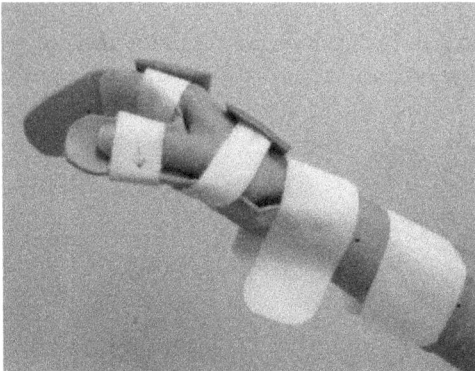

Fig. 2. Resting forearm splint.

Equipment for mobility

a. Lightweight, foldable, detachable wheelchair: these wheelchairs come with detachable armrests and footrests features which allow the wheelchair to be positioned next to the bed/commode/car seat to facilitate transfer. Large rear wheels (22–24 in) are for self-propulsion. Mid rear wheels (16–18 in) are easier for caregivers to manoeuvre. Recommended for individuals who need assistance with transfer

b. Lightweight, foldable, non-detachable wheelchair: these wheelchairs come with fixed armrests and footrests. Recommended for individuals who require supervision or are independent in transfers, but are unable to ambulate for approximately 50 m

c. Push chair/travel chair: these wheelchairs come with non-detachable features, and small rear wheels (8–10 inch). Recommended for individuals who require supervision or are independent in transfers and are able to ambulate for more than 50 m. Usually used for travelling as it is compact and light (for easy storage)

d. Customised wheelchair: these wheelchairs come with customised features to meet individual needs (e.g. lifestyle and environmental constraints). It is usually used by individuals with no/limited ambulation and are dependent on wheelchairs for their mobility and ADLs

e. Tilt-in-space wheelchair: these wheelchairs come with the power tilt (tilt-in-space) feature that allows the whole chair to tilt up to 30 or 60 degrees, while maintaining the hip and knee angles at 90 degrees. Tilt-in-space wheelchair (1) promotes proper seating alignment for individuals who cannot maintain pelvic, thoracic, or head position and/or balance against gravity for prolonged periods of time, (2) promotes thoracic extension and reduces the risk of respiratory and/or digestive complications, (3) provides a change in position without the risk of shear forces, (4) reduces the risk of skin breakdown by redistributing pressure from the pelvis to the back, and (5) provides appropriate position for individual who are at risk of postural hypotension

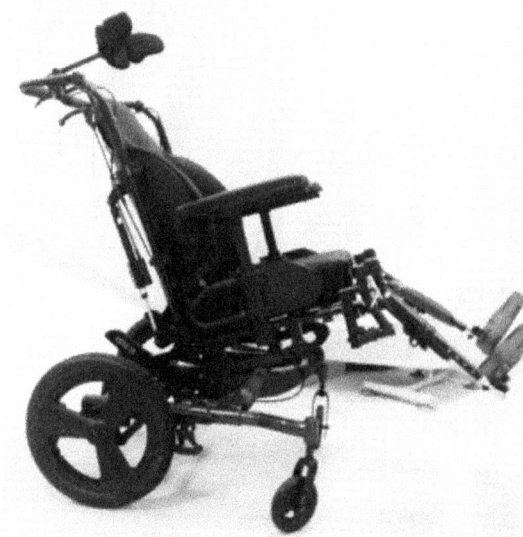

Fig. 3. Tilt-in-space wheelchair.

18
Rehabilitation Technology

LOH Yong Joo

Rehabilitation technology

- The systematic application of technologies, engineering methodologies, or scientific principles to meet the needs of, and address the barriers confronted by, individuals with disabilities in areas that includes education, rehabilitation, employment, transportation, independent living, and recreation. The term includes rehabilitation engineering, assistive technology devices, and assistive technology services

Rehabilitation engineering

- The systematic application of engineering sciences to design, develop, adapt, test, evaluate, apply, and distribute technological solutions to problems confronted by individuals with disabilities in functional areas, such as mobility, communications, hearing, vision, and cognition, and in activities associated with employment, independent living, education, and integration into the community

Assistive technology device

- Any item, piece of equipment or product system, whether acquired commercially, off the shelf, modified, or customise, that is used to increase, maintain, or improve the functional capabilities of an individual with a disability

Assistive technology service

- Any service that directly assists an individual in the selection, acquisition or use of an assistive technology device

Due to the numerous types of rehabilitation technologies available (and are always evolving due to advances), only the following commonly used clinical devices will be discussed.

Neuromuscular electrical stimulation (NMES)

- NMES refers to the process of applying electrical stimulation above the motor threshold to cause a muscle contraction. Successful use of NMES requires that the alpha motor neuron is intact. NMES systems utilises either external (most common) or internal electrodes to stimulate the muscle. NMES can be utilized as therapeutic muscle stimulation or for functional electrical stimulation

- External (most common): transcutaneous (surface) electrodes (frequencies of 10–50 Hz)

- Internal: implantable systems which use percutaneous, intramuscular, epineural, intraneural and intraspinal electrodes

- Therapeutic NMES: repetitive stimulation is applied to paralyzed muscles to minimise atrophy and/or maintain range of motion

- Functional electrical stimulation (FES): stimulation occurs in a coordinated sequence to assist the patient in performing a functional task, such as activities of daily living (ADLs), transfers, or ambulation. Employ either an open or closed loop system

- Open loop system
    - Feedback provided manually
    - Stimulation is activated by switches
    - Intensity is adjusted based on response
    - Example: therapist triggers a heel switch to activate anterior tibialis during gait cycle

- Closed loop system
    - More sophisticated system utilising more complex automated technology
    - Electrodes activated by computer generated patterns of stimulation to cause functional movements
    - Feedback is provided automatically through movement sensors
    - EMG-FES: EMG sensor triggers FES once threshold is reached; FES triggers desired movement
    - These systems are called neuroprostheses

- Examples:
  - ◆ Devices for foot drop: Ness L300, WalkAide
  - ◆ Devices used for upper limb function: Ness H200, Freehand system
  - ◆ Device for gait: Parastep system
- Clinical uses of NMES
  - Strengthens muscles and maintains muscle mass after immobilisation
  - Provides feedback to enhance voluntary muscle control
  - Provides cardiovascular conditioning (combine with FES cycle ergometer for patients with spinal cord injury)
  - Prevents complications from immobility, such as deep vein thrombosis, disuse atrophy, and osteoporosis
  - Shoulder subluxation in hemiplegic limb
- Precautions
  - Avoid stimulation over heart, neck, malignancies, pregnant uterus, or infected areas
  - May interfere with pacemakers
  - Caution with insensate skin (may cause burns)

Assistive technology devices

Assistive technology for communication disorders

- Commonly called augmentative and alternative communication (AAC) devices (Fig. 1)
  - Non-electronic systems: pictures from books or catalogues, using marker to draw letters/words/phrases/pictures
  - Electronic voice output systems (Digital Speech): to communicate quick, simple messages like "hi", "leave me alone" and can be activated both by direct or indirect selection (eye blink for locked in syndrome patients)
  - Portable amplification systems: for people who speak softly because of low breath support or other difficulties with phonation

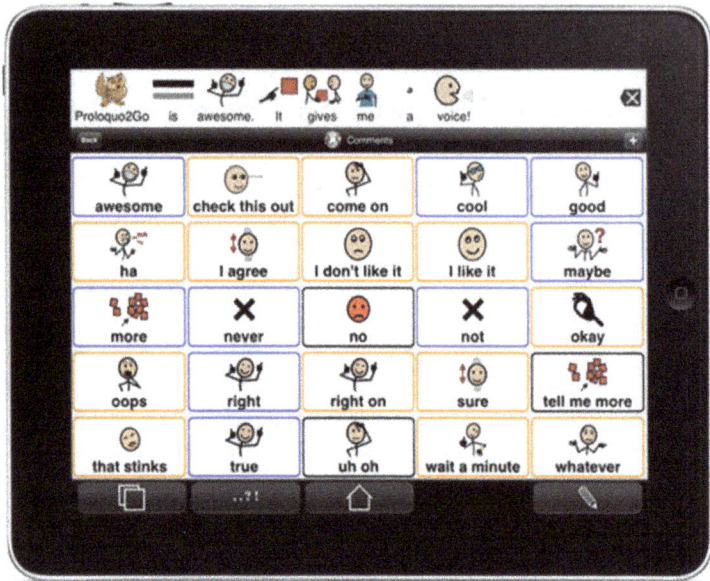

Fig. 1. AAC device.

Assistive technology for mobility impairments

- Upper body mobility devices
    - Alternate computer keyboards: expanded for difficulty in pointing accuracy, smaller keyboards designed for persons with limited range of motion and endurance
    - Voice recognition: writes by speaking words into a microphone
    - Onscreen keyboard: visible on computer monitor, wears a head-mounted signalling device or a reflective dot on the forehead to select keys on the onscreen keyboard
- Lower body mobility devices
    - Manual or powered wheelchair

Assistive technology for ergonomics and prevention of secondary injuries

- Growing area of concern is development of repetitive strain injuries (RSI)
- Deskbound jobs: properly supporting seated posture, raising or lowering a chair or desk for optimal fit, implementing routine breaks and using ergonomically designed keyboards

Electronic aids to daily living (EADL)

- Within the home, EADLs can control audio-visual equipment (e.g. television, video players and recorders, cable, digital satellite systems, and stereo), communication equipment (e.g. telephone, intercom, and call bells), doors, electric beds, security equipment, lights, and appliances (e.g. fan, and wave machine)

- EADLs are controlled directly by pressing a button with a finger or pointer or by voice command, or indirectly by scanning and switch activation

- Some AAC devices or computer systems also provide EADL control of devices within the environment

Assistive technology for hearing impairments

- Hearing aids

  - Used to facilitate both auditory input and speech output

  - Other types provide visual representation of the auditory signal (e.g. flashing lights as alternative emergency alarm)

  - Cochlear implants

  - Other hearing technologies

    - Computer assisted real-time translation

    - Involves a specially trained typist or stenographer who captures what is being spoken on a computer

Assistive technology for visual impairments

- Computers outfitted with a speech synthesiser and specialised software, allow navigation of the desktop, operating system, applications and documents, as well as the internet

- Portable note takers with either braille or speech synthesiser feedback for the user

- Screen magnification software for individuals with some degree of visual ability

Assistive technology for cognitive and learning disabilities

- Use of intelligent agents to interactively help people with everyday tasks in education, health care and workforce training

- Available on desktop or mobile computing devices

- Used to assist persons with cognitive disabilities to learn new job tasks or to prompt them through various steps within a task, or both

Rehabilitation robotics

Therapy robots

- Neurological: aims to help those born with little or non-existent neurological control by fostering or restoring muscle control
- Cardiopulmonary: for treatment of breathing problems and rehabilitation of individuals who have undergone cardiac trauma
- Musculoskeletal: enables individuals to restore functionality in the muscle group and skeleton by improving coordination and strength

Emotional and developmental therapy

- Shown to be beneficial to children and elderly individuals with a wide range of social, emotional and developmental disorders by creating a social engagement, promoting emotional response and motivating positive behaviour change
- Children with autism typically respond better and are drawn to computers and robots because of the predictable behaviour and reduced amount of external stimuli
- These robots mostly simulate a pet or a toy, and their main function is to increase user interaction, in a more or less intelligent manner, to enhance health and psychological well-being by providing companionship
- Some examples as follows:
  - Paro is a soft seal robot, and allows animal assistive therapy to be administered to patients. It is essentially targeted at the elderly in different environments and situations where live animals might pose treatment difficulties. Paro is not mobile, but it can be taught to act in a way that the user desires and stimulates interaction between patients and caregivers by responding to it. From interaction with humans, Paro responds by producing sounds, moving its head and legs and shows patient-favoured behaviour, thus giving the impression of a live animal. Paro has been proven to reduce stress or mental fatigue for patients, nurses and caregivers, improves the socialisation of patients with each other, increases their relaxation and motivation and enhances health and psychological well-being of the patients

Physical therapy

- Provides some form of physical support and mobility when the affected limb is no longer functional or has limitations

- 3 main categories: upper body extremities, lower body extremities and full body extremities

- Upper extremities: usually consists of arms with various degrees of freedom, where the position of the end effector is often represented graphically on a computer screen, whose endpoint is held by the patient's arm or hand. Normally divided into exoskeletal or end effector upper limb robotics

- Some examples as follows:

  - MIT-Manus (Fig. 2) provides high-intensity interactive physical therapy especially for stroke and spinal cord patients by improving movement of the shoulder, wrist and elbow on the affected side

  - Armeo is a highly responsive robot with a semi-exoskeleton or a full-exoskeleton structure with two passive and four active degrees of freedom, equipped with force and position sensors that allow naturalistic arm movement and shoulder translations to prevent joint degeneration and preserve joint mobility. The robot is equipped with an audio–visual display that detects movement and motivates the patient with simple games

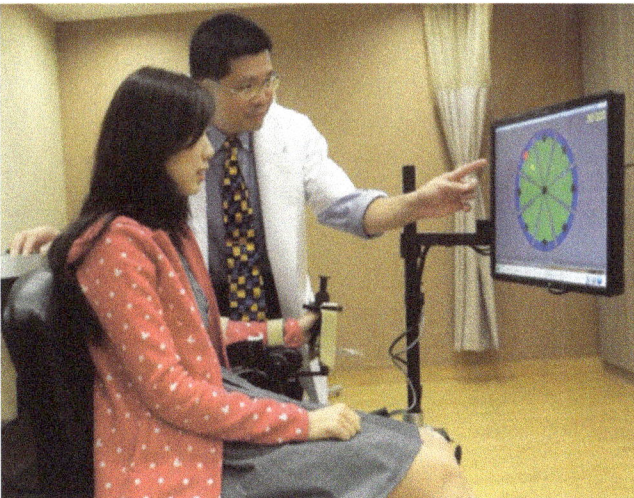

Fig. 2. MIT-Manus.

- Bi-Manu-track: one degree of freedom device designed for bilateral passive and active practice of forearm pronation/supination and wrist flexion/extension

- It has been shown that intensive and repetitive training combined with patient-compliant therapy can result in significant improvements in motor functions of the paretic arm even years after a stroke

- The rationale of using lower extremities robotics are as follows:

  - Longer and more intensive training sessions compared to manual treadmill

  - Provide real time feedback for a higher motivation and compliance

  - Physiological gait pattern provided by individually adjustable orthoses

  - Guidance force and body weight support, assessment and reporting functionality for an easy measurement of the patient's progress

  - Some examples:

    - Lokomat (Fig. 3) evidenced to reduce spasticity, improve walking ability, increase alertness, strengthen leg muscles, improve stamina and increase motivation

    - ReWalk: robot based on a patient's walking movements on the ground for gait training with a wearable brace support suit and backpack rechargeable batteries that integrate actuation motors at the joints, an array of motion sensors and an electronic and computer system with safety control and algorithms. ReWalk allows and helps a patient move as the centre of gravity shifts with their own control; this enables individuals with lower limb disabilities to perform routine ambulatory functions such as standing, walking and even climbing stairs

Virtual reality rehabilitation

- Definition of virtual reality (VR): computing technology that generates simulated or artificially three dimensional (3D) environment which imitates reality

- Classification: immersive, semi-immersive and non-immersive

- Immersive VR: user either uses a Head-Mounted Display (HMD), or a Head-Coupled Display (HCD) or be in a Cave Automatic Virtual

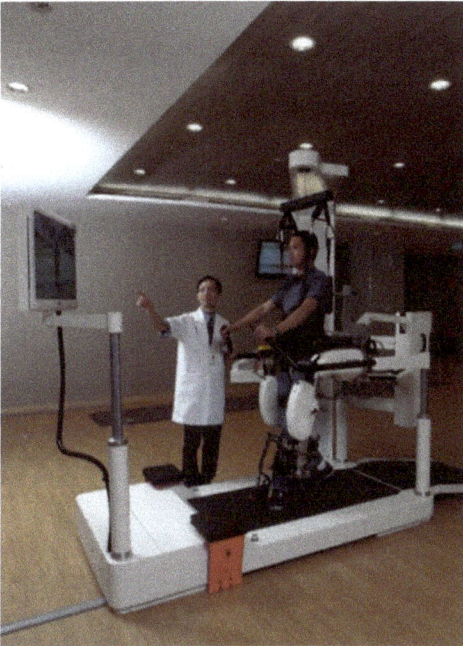

Fig. 3. Lokomat.

Environment (CAVE). Visual, auditory and tactile sensory aspects of the VE are delivered to the individual through visual display units and speakers within a HMD unit, data gloves, body suits or audio-visual systems in CAVE. Additional movement may be obtained using joystick, space ball, 3D mouse, other hand-held sensors, or cameras

- Non-immersive VR: user is placed in a 3D environment that can be directly manipulated with a conventional graphics workstation using a monitor, a keyboard or a mouse

- Semi-immersive VR: relatively high performance graphics computing system coupled with either a large screen monitor, large screen projector or multiple television projection systems. Using a wide field of view, semi-immersive system provides a better feeling of immersion or presence than non-immersive system

- Uses of VR
    - Medicine and healthcare to improve patient treatment and care
    - Rehabilitation: assessment, training, interaction and enablement
    - Memory training

- Improve lives of children with disabilities: improve quality of life, enhance social participation, improve life skills, mobility and cognitive abilities

- Advantages of VR rehabilitation
  - Safe and ecologically valid environments
  - Control over delivery of stimuli via adaptation of the environment and task to elicit various levels of performance
  - Gradual changes in task complexity while changing extent of therapist intervention
  - Increased standardisation of assessments and treatment protocols
  - Objective measurement of behaviour and performance
  - Provision of enjoyable and motivating experiences

- Examples of VR systems used:
  - Commercial off the shelf consoles: Nintendo Wii Sony PS3 with EyeToy, Microsoft Xbox with Kinect
  - Customized clinical systems: GestureTek IREX, SeeMe Rehab System, Mindmaze, Jintronix
  - VR for cognitive rehabilitation
  - Cognitive processes: visual and spatial perception, attention, memory, sequencing and executive functioning

- Attention
  - Virtual classroom for ADHD children assessment and rehabilitation
  - 2D IREX video-capture system to examine the feasibility of using VR for children with acquired brain injury

- Unilateral spatial neglect
  - Cancellation tasks, commonly used in rehabilitation clinics, can be manipulated via decreasing or increasing the size of the stimuli, can include cues to facilitate allocation of attention to the left space, or can measure hand movement during task performance

- Memory and spatial navigation
  - Potential to train individuals to improve their attention and memory abilities with a task that is relevant, similar to real-world settings,

but still controlled with the possibility of systematic and precise measurement

- Executive functions and dual tasking
    - Can readily be designed to simulate the demands found in everyday tasks
    - An example is VMall by GestureTek's GX VR platform
- Upper limb motor rehabilitation
    - VR to promote motor relearning for different movements (hand, elbow and shoulder) and functional tasks or goals
    - May be an effective and efficient approach to train a set of basic tasks with upgrading to a wide variety of skilled movements
- Lower limb motor rehabilitation
    - Designed to help recover efficient walking in patients with lower limb motor impairment after stroke
    - Usually with the use of walking aids, treadmill with or without body weight and robotics support

Recommended reading

- Cuccurullo S (Ed), Physical Medicine and Rehabilitation Board Review, 2nd ed. Demos Medical Publishing, New York, 2009.
- Selzer M, et al. (Eds). Textbook of Neural Repair and Rehabilitation, Medical Neurorehabilitation, Volume 2, 2nd ed. Cambridge University Press, Cambridge, 2014.
- Yakub F, et al. Recent trends for practical rehabilitation robotics, current challenges and the future. Int J Rehabil Res 2014;37(1):9–21.
- Brahnam S, Jain LC. Virtual reality in psychotherapy, rehabilitation and neurological assessment. Advanced Computational Intelligence Paradigms in Healthcare 6. Virtual Reality in Psychotherapy, Rehabilitation, and Assessment. Springer, Berlin Heidelberg, 2011, pp. 1–9.
- Laver K, et al. Cochrane review: virtual reality for stroke rehabilitation. Eur J Phys Rehabil Med. 2012;48(3):523–530.

19
Acupuncture in Rehabilitation

YEN Hwee Ling

What is acupuncture?

Acupuncture, as one of the prime modalities of Traditional Chinese Medicine (TCM), has been practised for more than 2,000 years. It involves the insertion of needles into specific points on the body to treat various illnesses. These acupuncture points can be found on meridians which run throughout the body. By accessing these points, the acupuncturist can influence the "qi" (energy) internally to achieve a smooth, unobstructed flow and to correct any deficiency or excess. This internal homeostasis is vital for good health. Selection of points for treatment is based on various TCM principles, such as yin-yang and the internal organs.

For the past few decades, a type of acupuncture practised by western medical doctors and allied health personnel has developed. This has been termed "medical acupuncture" and also involves the insertion of needles into specific points of the body. However, the selection of points is based on neuroanatomical and neurophysiological principles.

What are the scientific mechanisms behind the effectiveness of acupuncture?

The proposed mechanisms of acupuncture, especially in the treatment of pain, include:

- Release of endogenous opioid peptides
- Diffuse noxious inhibitory control
- Deactivation of trigger points

What does an acupuncture treatment session typically involve?

Based on the patient's history and physical findings, the acupuncturist formulates a diagnosis and selects the relevant acupuncture points. Which points are selected is based on the needs of the individual patient and may differ from one person to another even when they have the same condition. Needles are retained in the body for 20–30 minutes each time and patients often need more than one session. The time needed for benefits to be seen is highly variable and depends on the severity and chronicity of the underlying condition.

What are the side effects of acupuncture?

With properly trained acupuncturists using one-use disposable needles, the procedure is generally very safe. Side effects, if any, are mild and include local bleeding/bruising and transient pain around the needling site. Serious consequences, such as accidental trauma to underlying internal organs, are extremely rare.

What are the contraindications to acupuncture?

We do not advise needling areas with active skin lesions, such as ulcers or abscesses, or open wounds. Patients with serious bleeding disorders or who are on anticoagulation therapy should also not receive needling acupuncture. Those who have an implanted demand cardiac pacemaker should not have electro-acupuncture (in which low-level electrical currents are passed between the needles), to avoid interfering with the function of the pacemaker.

Is acupuncture effective?

To evaluate effectiveness, we have to analyse the outcome of acupuncture research. Unfortunately, in the field of acupuncture research, several major issues have been encountered. These include:

- It is not possible to do randomised double-blind placebo-controlled studies (the gold standard of medical research) as it is not possible to blind the acupuncturist

- There have been difficulties defining "sham" (fake) acupuncture as some studies appear to show that such sham acupuncture can also produce clinical effects

- Studies often involve heterogeneous groups of patients, making direct comparisons unreliable

- As this form of treatment has to be individualised in approach and point selection to be effective, a standardised regime cannot be applied to all patients

- Publication bias—research studies having "nil" or "negative" effects are much less likely to be published

Bearing these difficulties in mind, evidence in support of the efficacy of acupuncture, to date, is strongest in three types of conditions:

1. Chronic pain—such as neck and back pain, osteoarthritis, chronic headache

2. Postoperative nausea and vomiting

3. Postoperative pain

For the conditions commonly seen in the rehabilitation setting, such as stroke, spinal cord injury and traumatic brain injury, there has been no clear evidence that acupuncture is definitely beneficial.

What is the role of acupuncture in the rehabilitation setting?

In Singapore, there are several factors for acupuncture which include:

- Cultural factors—a significant proportion of the local population grew up with and accept TCM

- Acupuncture is deemed by the lay public to be safer than oral medicines, with fewer side effects

- The treatment approach is considered by some to be more personable

- There is a possibility of additional benefits over and above those seen with standard treatments (include pharmacological agents and rehabilitation)

If we were to be asked by patients and relatives about the usefulness of acupuncture, we would recommend adding acupuncture as complementary treatment to standard therapy in the following situation:

- Conditions: Apart from the three groups of conditions listed above, we would include acute neurological conditions (such as stroke and spinal cord injury); chronic conditions with recent flare or exacerbation (such as arthritis); pain which can be acute or chronic (particularly of musculoskeletal origin); and

- Patient and family are very keen

- Contraindications are absent

- The acupuncturist is qualified and experienced

We suggest a trial of 10–20 sessions initially to determine if acupuncture is beneficial.

Acknowledgment

"

This book would not have been possible without the administrative support and hard work by **Ms CHAN Sharon** and **Ms LIU Mengxi.**

"